PREFACE

The All-Inclusive Guide for Aspiring Professionals with Interactive T........ Job-Hunting Tactics is intended for those people with little to no knowledge in medical speciality, medical coding and billing or those already with knowledge but intend to revise or otherwise use it as a guidance in their daily practices.

The book starts with introduction to medical knowledge for those who are naïve to this filed, it goes further to give insights and instructions with vivid examples in coding and billing of commonly encountered specialities and sub specialities in medical fields, later on it delves into selected specialist with their nuances and inticacies

Furthermore, it explains and teaches how to tackle and pass examinations from the first day of examination preparation to the examination day, it also covers vital areas such as job hunting and how to pass interviews successfully.

Finally, there numerous exercises with their answers and explanation for why those answers are deemed correct.

Having read and participated in the preparation of this guidebook its my hope all medically naïve and those with some knowledge in this field will find this book indispensable whether its for the exampreparation or daily practices.

We welcome any suggestion, questions, corrections from readers as this will be assessed and incorporated in our upcoming versions of this guidebook.

Remigius Thadeo

Medical Doctor

Muhimbili National Hospital-Dar es Salaam

Medical Billing & Coding Mastery in 4 Months

© Copyright 2024 by Publishing Help

TABLE OF CONTENTS

INTRODUCTION

Medical billing and coding form the backbone of the healthcare revenue cycle, ensuring that healthcare providers are reimbursed for their services. This field requires a meticulous understanding of medical terminology, coding systems, and healthcare regulations. The journey to mastering medical billing and coding is both challenging and rewarding, offering a stable and lucrative career path for those who are dedicated. The healthcare system is a complex network of providers, patients, and payers, each playing a crucial role in delivering and financing care. Medical billers and coders act as intermediaries, translating patient encounters into standardized codes used for billing and statistical purposes. This process ensures accurate reimbursement and contributes to the healthcare system's overall efficiency and effectiveness.

Medical terminology is the language of healthcare, a specialized vocabulary used to describe the human body, its functions, diseases, and treatments. Understanding this language is essential for anyone involved in medical billing and coding. It allows professionals to interpret and code medical records accurately, ensuring the information is communicated clearly and consistently. Coding systems, such as the International Classification of Diseases (ICD) and the Current Procedural Terminology (CPT), provide a standardized way to classify and report medical diagnoses and procedures. These systems constantly evolve, reflecting advances in medical knowledge and changes in healthcare delivery. Staying current with these updates is a critical aspect of the job, requiring ongoing education and training.

Healthcare laws, ethics, and compliance are fundamental to medical billing and coding. Professionals in this field must adhere to strict regulations, such as the Health Insurance Portability and Accountability Act (HIPAA), which protects patient privacy and ensures the security of health information. Ethical considerations, such as accuracy and honesty in coding, are equally important, as they directly impact patient care and the financial health of healthcare providers. The roles of medical billers and coders are distinct yet interconnected. Billers are responsible for submitting claims to insurance companies and following up on unpaid claims, while coders assign the appropriate codes to diagnoses and procedures. Both roles require a keen eye for detail, strong analytical skills, and a thorough understanding of the healthcare system.

The medical billing and coding foundation is built on a solid understanding of the healthcare system, medical terminology, coding systems, and regulatory requirements. This knowledge is essential for accurately translating patient encounters into standardized codes, ensuring healthcare providers are reimbursed for their services. Medical terminology is the cornerstone of this field, providing the language needed to describe the human body, its functions, diseases, and treatments. With a firm grasp of this language, it is possible to interpret and code medical records accurately. Coding systems like ICD and CPT provide a standardized way to classify and report medical diagnoses and procedures. These systems constantly evolve, reflecting advances in medical knowledge and changes in healthcare delivery. Staying current with these updates is a critical aspect of the job, requiring ongoing education and training.

CHAPTER 1

FOUNDATIONS OF MEDICAL BILLING AND CODING

Overview of the Healthcare System

Healthcare systems around the world are intricate networks designed to provide medical services to populations. These systems vary widely in structure, funding, and delivery methods, reflecting different countries' diverse needs and resources. At their core, healthcare systems aim to promote health, prevent disease, and provide treatment for illnesses and injuries. Understanding these systems' fundamental components and functions is crucial for anyone entering the healthcare field or seeking to navigate their healthcare journey.

Healthcare systems can be broadly categorized into public, private, and private-public partnerships. The government typically funds and operates public healthcare systems, ensuring all citizens have access to essential medical services. These systems often emphasize preventive care and public health initiatives, aiming to reduce the overall disease burden on society. Examples of public healthcare systems include the National Health Service (NHS) in the United Kingdom and Medicare in Australia.

Private healthcare systems, on the other hand, are primarily funded through private insurance and out-of-pocket payments. These systems often offer higher personalized care and shorter wait times for services, but they can also be more expensive and less accessible to lower-income individuals. The United States is a notable example of a country with a predominantly private healthcare system, although it also has public programs like Medicare and Medicaid to support vulnerable populations. Private-public partnerships healthcare systems combine elements of both public and private systems, aiming to balance accessibility, quality, and cost. Countries like Canada and Germany have Private-public partnerships healthcare systems, where the government provides basic healthcare coverage, but individuals can also purchase private insurance for additional services or faster access to care. This hybrid approach seeks to leverage the public and private sectors' strengths while mitigating their weaknesses.

Several critical indicators, including life expectancy, infant mortality rates, and chronic disease prevalence, often measure a healthcare system's effectiveness. Additionally, factors such as patient satisfaction, access to care, and the efficiency of service delivery play a significant role in evaluating a system's performance. High-performing healthcare systems are characterized by their ability to provide timely, equitable, and high-quality care to all individuals, regardless of socio-economic status.

Various external factors influence healthcare systems, including economic conditions, political stability, and cultural attitudes towards health and wellness. For instance, countries with strong economies and stable governments are better equipped to invest in healthcare infrastructure and services. Conversely, nations facing economic challenges or political unrest may struggle to provide adequate healthcare to their populations, leading to disparities in healthcare provisions.

Technological advancements have also profoundly impacted healthcare systems, revolutionizing how medical services are delivered and managed. Innovations such as electronic health records (EHRs), telemedicine, and advanced diagnostic tools have improved the efficiency and accuracy of healthcare delivery, enabling providers to offer more personalized and effective care. However, integrating new technologies also presents challenges, including the need for significant investment, training, and regulatory oversight.

Healthcare systems are dynamic entities that must continuously adapt to changing needs and circumstances. For example, the COVID-19 pandemic has highlighted the importance of robust public health infrastructure and the need for flexible, responsive healthcare systems. Many countries have had to rapidly scale up their healthcare capacity, implement widespread testing and vaccination programs, and develop new protocols for managing infectious diseases. These experiences underscore the critical role of healthcare systems in safeguarding public health and responding to emerging threats.

In addition to addressing immediate health concerns, healthcare systems also play a vital role in promoting long-term health and wellness. Preventive care, health education, and community outreach programs are essential components of a comprehensive healthcare system, helping to reduce the incidence of chronic diseases and improve overall quality of life. Healthcare systems can enhance individual health outcomes and reduce the long-term costs of treating advanced illnesses by focusing on prevention and early intervention.

Healthcare systems are complex and multifaceted, encompassing various services, providers, and stakeholders. The healthcare professionals who deliver care are at the heart of these systems, including doctors, nurses, pharmacists, and allied health workers. These individuals are supported by a vast network of administrative staff, policy makers, and researchers who work together to ensure the smooth functioning of the system. Effective healthcare systems rely on strong leadership and governance to set priorities, allocate resources, and monitor performance. Policy makers play a crucial role in shaping healthcare systems and developing policies and regulations that promote access, quality, and sustainability. Collaboration between government agencies, private sector organizations, and non-profit entities is often necessary to address complex health challenges and achieve shared goals.

Healthcare systems are also shaped by the needs and preferences of the populations they serve. Patient-centred care, which prioritizes the needs and values of individuals, is increasingly recognized as a critical component of high-quality healthcare. This approach involves:

- Actively engaging patients in their care.
- Respecting their preferences.
- Providing personalized support and education.

By fostering solid patient-provider relationships and empowering individuals to take an active role in their health, healthcare systems can improve outcomes and enhance patient satisfaction.

Financing is another critical aspect of healthcare systems, determining how resources are generated, allocated, and utilized. Countries employ various financing models, each with advantages and disadvantages. In public healthcare systems, funding typically comes from taxation, ensuring that healthcare is accessible to all citizens. This model promotes equity but can be constrained by government budgets and economic fluctuations. In private systems, funding is often derived from private insurance premiums and out-of-pocket payments, which can lead to disparities in access and affordability. Private-public partnerships healthcare systems attempt to balance these approaches, combining public funding with private contributions to create a more comprehensive and flexible financing structure.

Healthcare systems must also navigate the complexities of cost control and resource allocation. Rising healthcare costs, driven by aging populations, technological advancements, and the increasing prevalence of chronic diseases, pose significant challenges for policymakers and providers.

Strategies to manage costs include implementing value-based care models, which focus on outcomes rather than volume of services, and promoting preventive care to reduce the need for expensive treatments.Additionally, healthcare systems may adopt price regulation, bulk purchasing, and negotiation with pharmaceutical companies to control costs and ensure the affordability of essential medications and services.

Workforce planning and development are essential components of a robust healthcare system. Ensuring an adequate supply of trained healthcare professionals is critical to meeting the population's needs and maintaining high standards of care. This involves recruiting and training new healthcare workers and retaining and supporting existing staff through continuing education, professional development opportunities, and measures to prevent burnout and improve job satisfaction. Addressing workforce shortages and imbalances, particularly in underserved areas, is a crucial priority for many healthcare systems.

Healthcare systems are also increasingly focused on addressing social determinants of health, recognizing that factors such as income, education, housing, and environment significantly shape health outcomes. By adopting a holistic approach that considers the broader context of individuals' lives, healthcare systems can more effectively address health disparities and promote overall well-being. This may involve partnerships with other sectors, such as education, housing, and social services, to develop integrated strategies addressing health inequities' root causes.

Patient safety and quality of care are paramount concerns for healthcare systems. Implementing evidence-based practices, adhering to clinical guidelines, and fostering a culture of continuous improvement are essential to ensuring that patients receive safe and effective care. Healthcare systems must also prioritize transparency and accountability, regularly monitoring performance and outcomes to identify areas for improvement and address any issues that arise. Engaging patients and families in safety initiatives and encouraging open communication can further enhance the quality of care and build trust in the healthcare system.

Innovation and research are driving forces behind the evolution of healthcare systems. Ongoing research and development efforts lead to new treatments, technologies, and approaches that can improve patient outcomes and enhance the efficiency of care delivery. Healthcare systems must be agile and open to adopting innovations while ensuring they are rigorously evaluated for safety, efficacy, and cost-effectiveness. Collaboration between academic institutions, industry, and healthcare providers is crucial to advancing medical research and translating discoveries into practical applications.

Global health challenges, such as pandemics, climate change, and antimicrobial resistance, underscore the interconnectedness of healthcare systems and the importance of international cooperation. Sharing knowledge, resources, and best practices across borders can enhance the ability of healthcare systems to respond to global threats and improve health outcomes worldwide. Organizations such as the World Health Organization (WHO) are crucial in coordinating international efforts and providing guidance and support to countries in strengthening their healthcare systems.

Healthcare systems continually evolve, shaped by a complex interplay of demographics, technology, policy, and societal values. As they adapt to new challenges and opportunities, the ultimate goal remains: to provide high-quality, accessible, and equitable care that promotes the health and well-being of all individuals. By understanding the intricacies of healthcare systems and the forces that influence them, stakeholders can work together to build a healthier future for everyone.

Introduction to Medical Terminology

Medical terminology forms the backbone of the healthcare industry, providing a universal language that enables precise communication among healthcare professionals. This specialized vocabulary is essential for accurately describing the human body, its functions, diseases, procedures, and treatments. Understanding medical terminology is crucial for anyone entering the healthcare field, as it ensures clarity and reduces the risk of errors in patient care. The language of medicine is built on a foundation of Latin and Greek roots, prefixes, and suffixes, which combine to create descriptive and specific terms. By mastering these components, healthcare professionals can communicate complex medical concepts quickly and precisely.

The origins of medical terminology can be traced back to ancient civilizations, where early physicians and scholars began to develop a systematic approach to describing the human body and its ailments. Latin and Greek were the languages of scholarship and science, and their influence is still evident in modern medical terminology. For example, the term "cardiology" is derived from the Greek word "kardia," meaning heart, and "logia," meaning study. Similarly, "dermatology" comes from the Greek word "derma," meaning skin, and "logia." This historical foundation provides a consistent and logical structure for medical terms, making them easier to learn and understand.

Medical terminology is not just a collection of obscure words but a dynamic and evolving language that adapts to medical discoveries and advancements. As medical knowledge expands so does new terms describe emerging diseases, technologies, and treatments. For instance, the advent of genetic testing and personalized medicine has introduced terms like "pharmacogenomics". Staying current with these developments is essential for healthcare professionals, ensuring they can accurately interpret and communicate the latest medical information.

Learning medical terminology can be challenging, but it is a skill that can be developed with practice and dedication. One practical approach is to break down complex terms into their parts—prefixes, roots, and suffixes—and understand their meanings. For example, the term "hypertension" can be dissected into "hyper," meaning excessive, and "tension," referring to pressure. By recognizing these building blocks, healthcare professionals can decipher unfamiliar terms and gain a deeper understanding of medical concepts. Additionally, using flashcards, mnemonic devices, and repetition can help reinforce this knowledge and improve retention.

Medical terminology is organized into several key categories, each focusing on different aspects of healthcare. These categories include anatomical terms, which describe the structure of the body; physiological terms, which explain the functions of organs and systems; pathological terms, which identify diseases and disorders; and procedural terms, which outline diagnostic and therapeutic interventions. Familiarity with these categories allows healthcare professionals to navigate the vast landscape of medical language and apply it effectively in their practice.

Anatomical terms are essential for accurately describing the human body and its regions. These terms often use directional and positional prefixes to specify the location of structures relative to one another. For example, "anterior" refers to the front of the body structure, while "posterior" denotes the back of the body structure. Similarly, "superior" indicates a position above, and "inferior" signifies a position below in relation to the body part being compared to. Understanding these terms is crucial for interpreting medical imaging, conducting physical examinations, and documenting patient findings.

Physiological terms describes the functions and processes of the body's organs and systems. These terms often incorporate prefixes and suffixes that indicate specific actions or conditions. For example, "bradycardia" combines "Brady," meaning slow with "cardia," referring to the heart, thus meaning a heart beating at a slower rate than normal. Similarly, "tachypnea" merges "tachy," meaning rapid, with "pnea," referring to breathing, to denote rapid breathing. Mastery of physiological terms enables healthcare professionals to accurately describe and assess bodily functions, facilitating effective diagnosis and treatment.

Pathological terms identify body diseases and disorders. These terms often include prefixes and suffixes that convey the nature and severity of the condition. For example, "osteoporosis" combines "osteo," meaning bone, with "porosis", indicating a porous or weakened state, to describe a condition characterized by porous and weak bones. Similarly, "hepatitis" merges "hepato," referring to the liver, with "itis," denoting inflammation, to describe inflammation of the liver. Recognizing pathological terms is essential for diagnosing and managing medical conditions and communicating with patients and colleagues.

Procedural terms outline diagnostic and therapeutic interventions used in healthcare. These terms often incorporate prefixes and suffixes that specify the type and purpose of the procedure. For example, "colonoscopy" combines "colon," referring to the colon, with "scope," meaning visual examination, to describe a procedure that involves examining the colon with a scope. Similarly, "angioplasty" merges "angio," meaning vessel, with "plasty," indicating moulding, to describe a procedure that involves widening narrowed blood vessels. Familiarity with procedural terms is crucial for understanding and performing medical interventions and documenting patient care.

Medical terminology is a living language, constantly evolving to keep pace with medical science and technology advancements. As new diseases emerge and innovative treatments are developed, the lexicon of medicine expands, incorporating terms that reflect these changes. For instance, the rise of telemedicine has introduced terms like "teleconsultation" and "telemonitoring," while advancements in robotics have given us "robot-assisted surgery." Keeping abreast of these developments is essential for healthcare professionals, ensuring they remain proficient in the latest terminology and can effectively communicate contemporary medical practices.

The importance of medical terminology extends beyond healthcare professionals to patients and their families. Clear and accurate communication is vital for patient education, informed consent, and shared decision-making. When healthcare providers use precise medical terms, they can explain diagnoses, treatment options, and prognoses more effectively, fostering a better understanding and trust between patients and providers. This transparency empowers patients to take an active role in their healthcare, improving outcomes and satisfaction.

Medical terminology also plays a critical role in medical documentation and record-keeping. Accurate and consistent terminology ensures that all healthcare team members understand patient records clearly, comprehensively, and efficiently. This is particularly important in complex cases where multiple specialists are involved, as it facilitates seamless communication and coordination of care. Moreover, standardized terminology is essential for coding and billing purposes, ensuring that healthcare services are accurately documented and reimbursed.

In the realm of medical research, terminology is indispensable for the dissemination of knowledge and the advancement of science. Researchers rely on precise and standardized language to describe their findings, enabling others to replicate studies, validate results, and build upon existing knowledge. Medical journals, conferences, and databases all depend on a shared vocabulary to facilitate the exchange of information and foster collaboration among scientists worldwide. By mastering medical terminology, researchers can contribute to the collective understanding of health and disease, driving innovation and progress in the field.

The study of medical terminology is not confined to textbooks and classrooms; it is a lifelong endeavour that requires continuous learning and adaptation. Healthcare professionals must stay current with new terms and concepts and refine their understanding of existing terminology. This ongoing education can be achieved through various means, such as attending conferences, participating in workshops, reading medical literature, and engaging in professional development activities. By committing to lifelong learning, healthcare professionals can maintain their proficiency in medical terminology and ensure they provide the highest standard of care.

In addition to formal education, practical experience is invaluable for mastering medical terminology. Hands-on training, clinical rotations, and real-world practice allow healthcare professionals to apply their knowledge in context, reinforcing their understanding and enhancing their skills. Interacting with patients, collaborating with colleagues, and navigating the healthcare environment contribute to a deeper and more intuitive grasp of medical language. This experimental learning is essential for developing the confidence and competence needed to communicate effectively in the fast-paced and dynamic world of healthcare.

Technology also plays a significant role in learning and applying medical terminology. Digital tools, such as online dictionaries, mobile apps, and electronic health records, provide convenient and accessible resources for healthcare professionals. These tools offer instant access to definitions, pronunciations, and examples, making learning and using medical terms easier. Additionally, technology can facilitate interactive learning experiences, such as virtual simulations which can enhance engagement and retention.

Integrating medical terminology into everyday practice is a testament to its importance and utility. From clinical documentation, research, and education, this specialized language permeates every aspect of healthcare. By mastering medical terminology, healthcare professionals can ensure clear and precise communication, improve patient care, and contribute to the advancement of medical science. This mastery is not merely an academic exercise but a practical and essential skill that underpins the entire healthcare system.

In conclusion, medical terminology is vital to healthcare, providing a universal language that enables precise and effective communication. Its historical roots in Latin and Greek and its dynamic and evolving nature make it a rich and complex field of study. By understanding and mastering medical terminology, healthcare professionals can enhance their ability to diagnose, treat, and educate, ultimately improving patient outcomes and advancing the field of medicine. The commitment to lifelong learning and practical application ensures that this essential skill remains sharp and relevant, supporting the ongoing mission of providing high-quality healthcare.

Coding Systems and Classifications

Coding systems and classifications form the backbone of modern healthcare, ensuring that medical information is accurately recorded, communicated, and analyzed. These systems provide a standardized language that allows healthcare professionals to consistently describe diagnoses, procedures, and other clinical information. This standardization is crucial for various aspects of healthcare, including patient care, billing, research, and public health surveillance. Without these systems, the complexity and volume of medical data would be overwhelming, leading to errors, inefficiencies, and compromising patient outcomes.

The origins of medical coding can be traced back to the early 20th century when the need for a systematic way to classify diseases and health conditions became apparent. The International Classification of Diseases (ICD) was one of the first coding systems developed, and it has since evolved through multiple revisions to accommodate new medical knowledge and practices. Today, the ICD is used worldwide, providing a common framework for reporting and monitoring diseases. Other coding systems, such as the Current Procedural Terminology (CPT) and the Healthcare Common Procedure Coding System (HCPCS), have been developed to classify medical procedures and services, further enhancing the precision and utility of medical coding.

Implementing coding systems and classifications has revolutionized healthcare by enabling more efficient and accurate documentation. For healthcare providers, these systems facilitate communication among multidisciplinary teams, ensuring that all members understand a patient's condition and treatment plan. This is particularly important in complex cases involving multiple specialists, as it helps coordinate care and avoid misunderstandings.

Additionally, standardized coding allows for more effective data analysis, enabling healthcare organizations to identify trends, measure outcomes, and improve the quality of care.

For patients, coding systems and classifications play a critical role in ensuring that their medical records are accurate and comprehensive. This accuracy is essential for continuity of care, as it allows new providers to quickly understand a patient's medical history and make informed decisions. Furthermore, standardized coding is vital for insurance, ensuring that claims are processed correctly and patients receive appropriate treatment coverage. By providing a clear and consistent way to document medical information, coding systems help to protect patients' rights and ensure that they receive the care they need.

In public health, coding systems and classifications are indispensable for monitoring and controlling diseases. By aggregating and analyzing coded data from various sources, public health authorities can track the spread of infectious diseases, identify emerging health threats, and evaluate the effectiveness of interventions. This information is crucial for developing evidence-based policies and allocating resources where needed. For example, during the COVID-19 pandemic, standardized coding allowed for rapid data collection and analysis, enabling public health officials to respond more effectively to the crisis.

The detailed explanation of coding systems and classifications reveals their complexity and the meticulous effort required to maintain and update them. The ICD, for instance, is currently in its 11th revision (ICD-11), which includes over 55,000 unique codes for diseases, conditions, and related health problems. Each code is structured hierarchically, with categories and subcategories that provide increasing levels of specificity. This hierarchical structure allows for broad and detailed analysis, making the ICD versatile for various applications.

Similarly, the CPT and HCPCS systems provide detailed medical procedures and service classifications. The CPT, maintained by the American Medical Association, includes codes for surgical procedures, diagnostic tests, and other medical services. Each code is accompanied by a description that specifies the procedure or service, ensuring that it is accurately documented and billed. The HCPCS, however, includes codes for products, supplies, and services not covered by the CPT, such as durable medical equipment and ambulance services. These systems provide a comprehensive framework for documenting and billing medical procedures.

Maintaining and updating coding systems continuously requires collaboration among healthcare professionals, researchers, and policymakers. New codes are added to reflect advancements in medical science, while outdated or redundant codes are revised or removed. This process ensures that coding systems remain relevant and accurate, supporting the evolving needs of the healthcare industry. Training and education are essential for ensuring that healthcare professionals use these systems proficiently. Many organizations offer certification programs and continuing education courses to help providers stay current with the latest coding practices.

The comprehensive review of coding systems and classifications highlights their impact on various aspects of healthcare. In clinical practice, these systems enhance the accuracy and efficiency of medical documentation, enabling providers to deliver high-quality care. For example, a physician diagnosing a patient with diabetes can use a specific ICD code to document the condition, ensuring that it is accurately recorded in the patient's medical record. This code can track the patient's progress, coordinate care with other providers, and submit insurance claims.

In medical research, coding systems provide a standardized way to collect and analyze data, facilitating the discovery of new insights and the development of innovative treatments. Researchers can use coded data to identify patterns and correlations, conduct epidemiological studies, and evaluate the effectiveness of interventions.

For instance, by analyzing ICD codes related to cardiovascular diseases, researchers can identify risk factors, track the prevalence of conditions, and assess the impact of lifestyle changes or medications on patient outcomes. This standardized data collection and analysis approach is essential for advancing medical knowledge and improving public health.

In healthcare administration, coding systems streamline the billing and reimbursement process, reducing errors and ensuring that providers are compensated accurately. Insurance companies rely on these codes to determine coverage and process claims, making it crucial for providers to use the correct codes to avoid delays or denials. Accurate coding also helps healthcare organizations manage their finances more effectively, providing a clear record of the services offered and the associated costs.

The role of coding systems in public health cannot be overstated. By providing a standardized way to report and monitor diseases, these systems enable public health authorities to track the spread of infectious diseases, identify emerging health threats, and evaluate the effectiveness of interventions. For example, public health officials can use ICD codes to quickly gather data on the number of cases, the geographic distribution, and the demographic characteristics of affected individuals during an outbreak of a new infectious disease. This information is crucial for developing targeted interventions and allocating resources where needed.

Integrating coding systems with electronic health records (EHRs) has enhanced their utility and efficiency. EHRs allow for the seamless capture, storage, and sharing of coded medical information, facilitating real-time access to patient data and improving care coordination. For instance, when patients visit a new healthcare provider, their EHR can be accessed to review their medical history, including diagnoses, procedures, and medications, all documented using standardized codes. This comprehensive view of the patient's health history enables providers to make informed decisions and deliver personalized care.

Moreover, using coding systems in EHRs supports population health management by enabling healthcare organizations to analyze data across large patient populations. This analysis can identify trends, measure outcomes, and develop strategies to improve the quality of care. For example, a healthcare organization might use coded data to identify patients with chronic conditions at risk of complications and develop targeted interventions to manage their care more effectively. By leveraging the power of coding systems and EHRs, healthcare organizations can enhance patient outcomes and reduce healthcare costs.

The future of coding systems and classifications in healthcare is likely to be shaped by advancements in technology and data analytics. Artificial intelligence (AI) and machine learning algorithms have the potential to revolutionize medical coding by automating the process and improving accuracy. These technologies can analyze vast amounts of data, identify patterns, and suggest the most appropriate codes, reducing the burden on healthcare providers and minimizing the risk of errors. Additionally, AI can support continuously updating and refining coding systems by identifying emerging trends and new medical knowledge.

Another promising development is integrating coding systems with other health information technologies, such as telemedicine and wearable devices. These technologies generate a wealth of data that can be coded and analyzed to provide insights into patient health and behaviour. For example, data from wearable devices that monitor physical activity, heart rate, and sleep patterns can be coded and integrated with EHRs to provide a more comprehensive view of a patient's health. This information can be used to develop personalized care plans and monitor the effectiveness of interventions in real time.

The global nature of healthcare and the increasing mobility of patients across borders also highlight the importance of standardized coding systems. International collaboration and harmonization of coding standards are essential to ensure that medical information can be accurately exchanged and understood across different healthcare systems. Organizations like the World Health Organization (WHO) are crucial in developing and promoting international coding standards, such as the ICD, to facilitate global health communication and cooperation.

In conclusion, coding systems and classifications are:

- Indispensable tools in modern healthcare.
- Are used to provide a standardized language for documentation.
- Are used for analyzing data.
- Are used to communicate medical information.

Their impact is felt across various aspects of healthcare, from clinical practice and research to public health and administration. These systems will become even more efficient and accurate as technology advances, supporting high-quality care and advancing medical knowledge. The ongoing collaboration among healthcare professionals, researchers, and policymakers will be essential to ensure that coding systems remain relevant and effective in meeting the needs of the healthcare industry.

Healthcare Laws, Ethics and Compliance

Healthcare laws, ethics, and compliance form the backbone of the medical industry, ensuring that patient care is delivered in a manner that is both legally sound and morally upright. These elements are crucial for maintaining trust between patients and healthcare providers, safeguarding patient rights, and ensuring that medical practices adhere to established standards. Understanding these components is essential for anyone involved in the healthcare sector, from administrators to practitioners, as they navigate the complex landscape of medical care.

Healthcare laws encompass a wide range of regulations and statutes designed to protect patient safety, ensure the quality of care, and regulate the operations of healthcare facilities. These laws address issues such as patient privacy, informed consent, and the licensing and accreditation of healthcare providers. For instance, the Health Insurance Portability and Accountability Act (HIPAA) in the United States sets stringent standards for protecting patient health information, ensuring that personal data is kept confidential and secure. Similarly, laws governing medical malpractice establish the legal framework for addressing instances of negligence or substandard care, providing a mechanism for patients to seek redress and hold providers accountable.

Ethics in healthcare involves the application of moral principles to medical practice, guiding the behavior and decision-making of healthcare professionals. Ethical considerations in healthcare are multifaceted, encompassing patient autonomy, beneficence, non-maleficence, and justice. Patient autonomy refers to the right of individuals to make informed decisions about their healthcare, free from coercion or undue influence. Beneficence and non-maleficence, on the other hand, require healthcare providers to act in the best interests of their patients, promoting their well-being while avoiding harm. Justice in healthcare ethics involves ensuring that resources are distributed fairly and that all patients receive equitable treatment, regardless of their background or circumstances.

Compliance in healthcare refers to the adherence to laws, regulations, and ethical standards that govern medical practice. This involves implementing policies and procedures to ensure that healthcare organizations and providers operate within the legal and moral framework established by regulatory bodies. Compliance programs are essential for identifying and mitigating risks, preventing fraud and abuse, and promoting a culture of accountability and transparency. Effective compliance programs typically include regular training and education for staff, robust reporting and monitoring systems, and mechanisms for addressing violations and enforcing corrective actions.

Healthcare laws, ethics, and compliance interplay are complex and dynamic, requiring continuous attention and adaptation. For example, advances in medical technology and societal values can lead to new ethical dilemmas and necessitate updates to existing laws and regulations. Healthcare providers must stay informed about these developments and be prepared to adjust their practices accordingly. This requires a commitment to ongoing education and professional development and a willingness to engage in open dialogue and collaboration with colleagues, patients, and regulatory authorities.

One of the critical challenges in healthcare law and ethics is balancing individual patients' rights and interests with society's broader needs. For instance, public health initiatives like vaccination programs and quarantine measures may conflict with personal autonomy and privacy rights. In such cases, healthcare providers must carefully weigh the potential benefits and harms, considering the ethical principles and legal requirements. This often involves difficult decisions and trade-offs, highlighting the importance of moral reasoning and sound judgment in medical practice.

Another important aspect of healthcare compliance is the prevention of fraud and abuse. Fraudulent activities, such as billing for services not rendered or falsifying patient records, undermine the healthcare system's integrity and divert valuable resources from patient care. Compliance programs are crucial in detecting and preventing such activities, ensuring that healthcare providers operate honestly and honestly. This requires a proactive approach, including regular audits and inspections, clear communication of expectations and standards, and a solid commitment to ethical behavior at all levels of the organization.

Healthcare laws, ethics, and compliance are not static; they evolve in response to new challenges and opportunities. For example, the rise of telemedicine and digital health technologies has introduced new ethical and legal considerations, such as ensuring patient privacy and data security in virtual consultations. Similarly, the increasing focus on patient-centered care and shared decision-making has highlighted the importance of respecting patient autonomy and involving patients in their care decisions. Healthcare providers must adapt and respond to these changes, continuously updating their knowledge and practices to stay current with the latest developments.

In addition to legal and ethical considerations, healthcare compliance involves adhering to industry standards and best practices. This includes following guidelines and recommendations from professional organizations, such as the American Medical Association (AMA) or the World Health Organization (WHO), and complying with accreditation requirements from bodies such as The Joint Commission. By aligning their practices with these standards, healthcare providers can ensure that they deliver high-quality care and meet the expectations of patients, regulators, and other stakeholders.

Effective communication is a critical component of healthcare compliance. This involves transparent, accurate patient care documentation, open and honest communication with patients, families, and colleagues. Transparency and accountability are essential for building trust and maintaining the integrity of the healthcare system. Healthcare providers must be willing to listen to feedback, address concerns, and take responsibility for their actions. This fosters a culture of trust and collaboration, essential for delivering high-quality care and ensuring patient satisfaction.

Regarding patient privacy, healthcare providers must balance sharing necessary information for patient care and protecting sensitive data. The advent of electronic health records (EHRs) has streamlined the sharing of patient information among healthcare providers. Still, it has also introduced new risks related to data breaches and unauthorized access. Ensuring compliance with privacy laws such as HIPAA requires robust security measures, regular staff training, and a vigilant approach to monitoring and addressing potential vulnerabilities.

Informed consent is another critical aspect of healthcare ethics and compliance. Patients have the right to be fully informed about their treatment options, including the potential risks and benefits, before making decisions about their care. This requires healthcare providers to communicate clearly and effectively, ensuring that patients understand the information and can ask questions.

Informed consent is not just a legal requirement; it is a fundamental ethical principle that respects patient autonomy and promotes trust in the patient-provider relationship.

Healthcare providers must also be mindful of cultural and linguistic diversity when obtaining informed consent and delivering care. This involves being aware of and sensitive to patient's cultural beliefs and practices and providing language assistance services when needed. By fostering an inclusive and respectful environment, healthcare providers can ensure that all patients receive equitable care and feel valued and understood.

The role of healthcare administrators in ensuring compliance cannot be overstated. Administrators are responsible for developing and implementing policies and procedures that align with legal and ethical standards and overseeing healthcare facilities' day-to-day operations. This includes conducting regular audits and assessments to identify areas of non-compliance, providing ongoing training and education for staff, and addressing any issues that arise promptly and effectively. Strong leadership and a commitment to ethical behavior are essential for creating a culture of compliance and accountability within healthcare organizations.

Healthcare laws, ethics, and compliance are interconnected and mutually reinforcing. Adhering to legal requirements helps uphold ethical principles, while a solid moral foundation supports compliance with laws and regulations. Together, they create a framework for delivering high-quality, patient-centered care that respects the rights and dignity of all individuals.

In the ever-evolving landscape of healthcare, staying informed and adaptable is crucial. Healthcare providers must proactively seek new knowledge and skills, stay current with changes in laws and regulations, and continuously reflect on their ethical responsibilities. This requires a commitment to lifelong learning and professional development and a willingness to engage in open dialogue and collaboration with colleagues, patients, and regulatory authorities.

Ultimately, healthcare laws, ethics, and compliance ensure patients receive safe, effective, and compassionate care. By adhering to these principles, healthcare providers can build trust with their patients, uphold the integrity of the healthcare system, and contribute to society's overall well-being.

The Roles of Medical Billers and Coders

Medical billers and coders play pivotal roles in the healthcare industry as the bridge between healthcare providers, patients, and insurance companies. Their work ensures that healthcare services are accurately documented and appropriately billed, which is essential for the financial health of medical practices and the overall efficiency of the healthcare system. These professionals must possess a keen eye for detail, a thorough understanding of medical terminology, and a firm grasp of coding systems and billing procedures.

Medical coders are responsible for translating the services provided by healthcare professionals into standardized codes. These codes communicate with insurance companies and other payers, ensuring that providers are reimbursed for their services. Coders must be proficient in various coding systems, such as the International Classification of Diseases (ICD) and the Current Procedural Terminology (CPT). They must also stay up-to-date with changes in coding guidelines and regulations, as these can impact the accuracy and efficiency of the billing process.

On the other hand, medical billers are responsible for submitting claims to insurance companies and following up on unpaid claims. They must ensure that claims are accurate and complete, as errors can lead to delays in payment or denials. Billers must also be familiar with the policies and procedures of insurance companies and government programs like Medicare and Medicaid. In addition to submitting claims, billers often handle patient billing inquiries, process payments, and manage accounts receivable.

The roles of medical billers and coders are closely intertwined, and effective communication between these professionals is crucial. Coders must provide accurate and detailed information to billers, who then use this information to submit claims and secure payment. Any discrepancies or errors in coding can lead to issues with billing, which can ultimately impact the financial stability of a healthcare practice. Therefore, billers and coders must work diligently to ensure their work is precise and thorough.

Medical billers and coders must also navigate the complexities of healthcare regulations and compliance. They must adhere to guidelines set forth by organizations such as the Centers for Medicare & Medicaid Services (CMS) and the Health Insurance Portability and Accountability Act (HIPAA). Compliance with these regulations is essential for protecting patient privacy and ensuring that billing practices are ethical and legal. This requires ongoing education and training, as well as a commitment to staying informed about changes in the regulatory landscape.

In addition to their technical skills, medical billers and coders must possess strong organizational and time management abilities. They often handle large volumes of information and must be able to prioritize tasks effectively. Attention to detail is critical, as even minor errors can have significant consequences. For example, an incorrect code can lead to a claim being denied, delaying payment and creating additional work for billers and coders. Therefore, these professionals must be meticulous and strive for accuracy in all aspects of their job.

Medical billers and coders also play a crucial role in ensuring patients receive the necessary care. By accurately documenting services and submitting claims promptly, they help to secure the required financial resources for healthcare providers to continue offering high-quality care. This, in turn, supports the overall health and well-being of patients. In some cases, billers and coders may also assist patients with understanding their bills and navigating the complexities of insurance coverage, providing valuable support and guidance.

The demand for skilled medical billers and coders is expected to grow in the coming years, driven by an ageing population and the increasing complexity of healthcare services. As the healthcare industry evolves, these professionals must adapt to new technologies and processes. For example, adopting electronic health records (EHRs) has transformed how medical information is documented and shared, requiring billers and coders to become proficient in using these systems. Additionally, advancements in medical treatments and procedures will necessitate ongoing education and training to ensure that coding and billing practices remain current and accurate.

Medical billers and coders must also be prepared to handle the challenges of their roles. This includes managing the stress of working in a fast-paced environment, dealing with complex and sometimes ambiguous information, and navigating the intricacies of insurance policies and regulations. Practical problem-solving skills are essential, as billers and coders must often identify and resolve issues related to claims and billing. This requires analytical thinking, attention to detail, and strong communication skills.

Despite the challenges, a medical billing and coding career can be gratifying. These professionals play a vital role in the healthcare system, contributing to the financial stability of medical practices and ensuring that patients receive the care they need. The work of billers and coders is essential for maintaining the integrity and efficiency of the healthcare industry, and their efforts directly impact the lives of patients and healthcare providers alike.

Medical billers and coders must also use technology to streamline their work. This includes proficiency with billing software, coding tools, and electronic health records (EHR) systems. Technology can help to automate many aspects of the billing and coding process, reducing the risk of errors and improving efficiency. However, billers and coders must stay current with technological advancements and continuously update their skills. This ongoing learning process is crucial for maintaining accuracy and staying competitive.

Integrating artificial intelligence (AI) and machine learning into medical billing and coding is another significant development. These technologies can analyze vast amounts of data quickly and accurately, identifying patterns and potential errors that human coders might miss. While AI can enhance the efficiency and accuracy of billing and coding, it also necessitates that professionals in the field understand how to work alongside these technologies, leveraging their capabilities while maintaining oversight to ensure that the human element of judgment and decision-making is not lost.

Medical billers and coders must also be prepared to adapt to healthcare policy and regulations changes. For instance, shifts in government healthcare programs, such as updates to Medicare and Medicaid, can have significant implications for billing practices. Staying informed about these changes and understanding their impact on coding and billing is essential for compliance and accuracy. This requires a proactive approach to professional development, including attending workshops, participating in continuing education courses, and staying connected with professional organizations.

Effective communication is another critical skill for medical billers and coders. They must clearly and accurately convey information to healthcare providers, insurance companies, and patients. This includes explaining complex billing issues, resolving discrepancies, and providing guidance on insurance coverage. Strong communication skills help build trust and ensure all parties understand the billing process clearly.

The role of medical billers and coders extends beyond the technical aspects of their job. They also contribute to the overall patient experience by ensuring that billing processes are smooth and transparent. By providing clear and accurate billing information, they help to alleviate some of the stress and confusion that patients may experience when dealing with medical bills. This, in turn, supports a positive relationship between patients and healthcare providers.

Medical billers and coders often work in various settings, including hospitals, clinics, private practices, and billing companies. Each of these environments presents unique challenges and opportunities. For example, working in a hospital setting may involve handling more claims and complex cases, while working in private practice may offer a more focused and specialized experience. Regardless of the setting, medical billers' and coders' core skills and responsibilities remain consistent.

The career path for medical billers and coders can also offer opportunities for advancement. With experience and additional training, professionals in this field can move into supervisory or management roles, overseeing teams of billers and coders. They may also choose to specialize in a particular coding area, such as oncology or cardiology, which can enhance their expertise and marketability. Additionally, some billers and coders may pursue roles in healthcare administration or consulting, leveraging their billing and coding knowledge to improve processes and systems within healthcare organizations.

The importance of ethical practices in medical billing and coding cannot be overstated. Adhering to ethical standards ensures that billing practices are fair, transparent, and compliant with regulations. This includes accurately representing services, avoiding fraudulent billing practices, and protecting patient privacy. Ethical behavior is essential for maintaining the trust of patients, healthcare providers, and insurance companies, and it supports the overall integrity of the healthcare system.

Medical billers and coders must also be prepared to handle sensitive and confidential information. This includes patient medical records, insurance details, and financial information. Protecting this information is a critical aspect of their role, and it requires a thorough understanding of privacy regulations, such as HIPAA. Ensuring patient information is handled with care and confidentiality is essential for maintaining trust and compliance.

In summary, medical billers and coders play a vital role in the healthcare industry, ensuring services are accurately documented and appropriately billed. Their work supports the financial health of medical practices, facilitates the reimbursement process, and contributes to the overall efficiency of the healthcare system. By staying current with coding guidelines, regulations, and technological advancements, these professionals can continue to provide valuable support to healthcare providers and patients. Their dedication to accuracy, ethical practices, and ongoing professional development is essential for maintaining the integrity and effectiveness of the billing and coding process.

Chapter Review with Interactive Exercises

Introduction to Medical Billing and Coding

Review: Medical billing and coding form the backbone of the healthcare revenue cycle. This subchapter introduces the fundamental concepts, including the roles and responsibilities of medical billers and coders, the importance of accuracy, and their impact on healthcare providers and patients.

Interactive Exercise:

Role Identification: List three critical responsibilities of a medical biller and three key responsibilities of a medical coder. Compare and contrast these roles.

Impact Analysis: Write a short paragraph on how accurate medical billing and coding can affect patient care and healthcare providers.

Understanding Coding Systems

Review: This subchapter delves into the various coding systems used in medical billing, such as ICD-10, CPT, and HCPCS. It explains the purpose of each system and how they are used to classify diagnoses, procedures, and services.

Interactive Exercise:

Coding Practice: Given a list of medical procedures and diagnoses, assign the appropriate ICD-10 and CPT codes.

System Comparison: Create a Venn diagram comparing ICD-10, CPT, and HCPCS codes, highlighting their unique and overlapping features.

The Billing Process

Review: The billing process involves several steps, from patient registration to claim submission and payment posting. This subchapter outlines each step in detail, emphasizing the importance of accuracy and timeliness.

Interactive Exercise:

Process Mapping: Draw a flowchart of the medical billing process, including all critical steps and decision points.

Scenario Analysis: Given a hypothetical patient visit, outline the billing process from start to finish, identifying potential challenges and solutions.

Ethical Standards and Compliance

Review: Ethical behavior and compliance with regulations are crucial in medical billing and coding. This subchapter covers vital ethical principles, common compliance issues, and consequences of non-compliance.

Interactive Exercise:

Ethical Dilemmas: Present a series of moral dilemmas related to medical billing and coding. Discuss how you would handle each situation.

Compliance Checklist: Create a checklist of compliance requirements for medical billers and coders, including critical regulations and best practices.

Technology in Medical Billing and Coding

Review: Technology plays a significant role in modern medical billing and coding. This subchapter explores the use of electronic health records (EHR) systems, billing software, and other digital tools that streamline the billing process and improve accuracy.

Interactive Exercise:

Tech Tools: Research and list five popular EHR systems or billing software used in the industry. Describe their key features and benefits.

Simulation: Use a demo version of an EHR system to practice entering patient information and generating a billing claim.

Continuing Education and Professional Development

Review: Continuing education and professional development are essential for staying current in the ever-evolving medical billing and coding field. This subchapter highlights the importance of ongoing learning, certification programs, and networking opportunities.

Interactive Exercise:

Certification Pathways: Research and outline the steps to obtain a Certified Professional Coder (CPC) or Certified Coding Specialist (CCS) certification.

Professional Development Plan: Create a personal, professional development plan, including goals, resources, and a timeline for achieving them.

CHAPTER 2

MASTERING MEDICAL TERMINOLOGY

Prefixes, Suffixes and Root Words

Understanding the building blocks of medical terminology is essential for anyone entering the field of medical billing and coding. Prefixes, suffixes, and root words form the foundation of this specialized language, enabling professionals to decipher complex terms and ensure accurate documentation. These components facilitate communication among healthcare providers and play a crucial role in the billing process, where precision is paramount.

Imagine a scenario where a patient visits a clinic complaining of chest pain. The physician documents the diagnosis as "angina pectoris." For a medical coder, recognizing that "angina" refers to chest pain and "pectoris" pertains to the chest is crucial for assigning the correct code. This understanding stems from a solid grasp of prefixes, suffixes, and root words. By breaking down medical terms into these components, coders can accurately interpret and code diagnoses and procedures, ensuring that healthcare providers are reimbursed correctly and patients receive appropriate care.

Prefixes are the initial components of medical terms, often indicating location, time, number, or status. For instance, the prefix "hyper-" means excessive or above average, as seen in "hypertension" (high blood pressure). Conversely, "hypo-" signifies below average, as in "hypoglycemia" (low blood sugar). Recognizing these prefixes allows coders to quickly grasp the context of a term, streamlining the coding process.

Suffixes, found at the end of medical terms, typically denote procedures, conditions, or diseases. For example, "-ectomy" means surgical removal, as in "appendectomy" (removal of the appendix), while "-itis" indicates inflammation, as in "arthritis" (inflammation of the joints). Understanding suffixes helps coders identify the nature of a medical term, ensuring accurate documentation and coding.

Root words form the core of medical terms, providing the primary meaning. These roots often derive from Latin or Greek, reflecting the historical development of medical language. For instance, "cardi-" refers to the heart, as seen in "cardiology" (the study of the heart), while "derm-" pertains to the skin, as in "dermatology" (the study of the skin). By recognizing root words, coders can decipher the fundamental meaning of medical terms, facilitating accurate coding and billing.

Consider the term "gastroenteritis." Breaking it down, "gastro-" refers to the stomach, "entero--" pertains to the intestines, and "-itis" indicates inflammation. Thus, "gastroenteritis" means inflammation of the stomach and intestines. This ability to deconstruct medical terms is invaluable for coders, enabling them to assign precise codes and ensure accurate billing.

The importance of mastering prefixes, suffixes, and root words extends beyond coding accuracy. It also enhances communication among healthcare providers, fostering a shared understanding of medical terminology. This shared language is crucial in a field where precision and clarity are vital. For instance, when a physician documents a diagnosis of "myocardial infarction," a coder who understands that "myo-" refers to muscle, "cardi-" pertains to the heart, and "infarction" means tissue death can accurately code the term as a heart attack. This accuracy ensures that the patient's medical record is clear and that the healthcare provider is reimbursed appropriately.

To further illustrate the significance of these components, consider the term "nephrectomy." By recognizing that "nephro-" refers to the kidney and "-ectomy" means surgical removal, a coder can accurately interpret the term as the surgical removal of a kidney. This understanding is crucial for accurately assigning the correct code and documenting the procedure.

Mastering prefixes, suffixes, and root words also aids in understanding medical abbreviations, which are commonly used in healthcare documentation. For example, "CABG" stands for coronary artery bypass graft, a procedure to improve blood flow to the heart. By breaking down the abbreviation, coders can accurately interpret and code the procedure, ensuring proper documentation and billing.

In addition to enhancing coding accuracy, a solid grasp of medical terminology can improve job performance and career advancement. Employers value coders who can accurately interpret and code medical terms, as this skill directly impacts the revenue cycle and patient care. By mastering prefixes, suffixes, and root words, coders can demonstrate their expertise and contribute to the efficiency and accuracy of the billing process.

To reinforce this knowledge, consider engaging in interactive exercises that challenge your understanding of medical terminology. For instance, practice breaking down complex medical terms into their components and assigning the appropriate codes. This hands-on approach can solidify your knowledge and improve your coding accuracy.

Another effective strategy is to create flashcards with common prefixes, suffixes, and root words. Reviewing these flashcards can help reinforce your knowledge and improve your ability to interpret medical terms quickly and accurately. Additionally, consider joining study groups or online forums where you can discuss medical terminology with peers and share tips and strategies for mastering this essential skill.

In summary, mastering prefixes, suffixes, and root words is crucial for anyone entering the field of medical billing and coding. This foundational knowledge not only enhances coding accuracy but also improves communication among healthcare providers and contributes to the overall efficiency of the billing process. By breaking down complex medical terms into their components, coders can accurately interpret and code diagnoses and procedures, ensuring that healthcare providers are reimbursed correctly and patients receive appropriate care.

Consider the term "osteoporosis." By recognizing that "osteo-" refers to bone and "-porosis" indicates a condition of porousness, a coder can accurately interpret the term as a condition characterized by weakened bones. This understanding is crucial for assigning the correct code and documenting the diagnosis accurately.

Another example is the term "electrocardiogram." Breaking it down, "electro-" refers to electricity, "cardio-" pertains to the heart, and "-gram" means a recording or a written record. Thus, an electrocardiogram records the electrical activity of the heart. This ability to deconstruct medical terms is invaluable for coders, enabling them to assign precise codes and ensure accurate billing.

The significance of mastering medical terminology extends to understanding procedural terms as well. For instance, "laparoscopy" combines "laparo-" (referring to the abdominal wall) and "-scopy" (meaning to view or examine). This term describes a minimally invasive surgical procedure used to analyze the organs inside the abdomen. By understanding the components of the term, coders can accurately interpret and code the procedure, ensuring proper documentation and billing.

Understanding medical terminology also aids in recognizing and interpreting medical abbreviations commonly used in healthcare documentation. For example, "COPD" stands for chronic obstructive pulmonary disease, a condition characterized by chronic obstruction of lung airflow. By breaking down the abbreviations, coders can accurately interpret and code the conditions, ensuring proper documentation and billing.

In the realm of medical billing and coding, precision is paramount. A single error in coding can lead to claim denials, delayed payments, and potential legal issues. By mastering prefixes, suffixes, and root words, coders can minimize errors and ensure that medical records are accurate and complete. This attention to detail benefits healthcare providers and enhances patient care by ensuring that diagnoses and treatments are accurately documented.

Consider the term "hepatomegaly." By recognizing that "hepato-" refers to the liver and "-megaly" indicates enlargement, a coder can accurately interpret the term as an enlarged liver. This understanding is crucial for assigning the correct code and documenting the diagnosis accurately.

Body Systems

The human body is a marvel of biological engineering, a complex network of systems working harmoniously to sustain life. Each system, from the circulatory to the nervous, plays a crucial role in maintaining homeostasis and ensuring that the body functions optimally. Understanding these systems is fundamental to grasping how our bodies operate and respond to various stimuli. The intricate interplay between these systems highlights the sophistication of human physiology and underscores the importance of maintaining a healthy lifestyle to support their functions.

The circulatory system, often called the body's transportation network, delivers oxygen and nutrients to cells while removing waste products. The heart, a muscular organ, pumps blood through a vast network of arteries, veins, and capillaries. This system sustains cellular metabolism and regulates body temperature and pH balance. The efficiency of the circulatory system is vital for overall health, as any disruption can lead to severe conditions such as hypertension, atherosclerosis, or heart failure.

The respiratory system works with the circulatory system to ensure that oxygen reaches the bloodstream and carbon dioxide is excreted from the body. The lungs, the primary organs of this system, facilitate gas exchange through tiny air sacs called alveoli. Breathing, an involuntary yet essential process, is controlled by the medulla oblangata. Proper respiratory function is crucial for maintaining oxygen levels and ensuring that metabolic processes proceed without interruption.

The digestive system is another critical component that breaks down food into nutrients that the body can absorb and utilize. This system includes the mouth, oesophagus, stomach, intestines, gallbladder, liver, and pancreas. Each organ plays a specific role in digestion and absorption, from mechanical breakdown in the mouth to chemical digestion in the stomach and nutrient absorption in the intestines. The liver, gallbladder and pancreas contribute by producing bile and digestive enzymes. A well-functioning digestive system is essential for energy production, growth, and repair.

The nervous system, comprising the brain, spinal cord, and peripheral nerves, acts as the body's control centre. It processes sensory information, coordinates voluntary and involuntary actions, and facilitates communication between body parts. The brain is a highly complex organ responsible for cognitive functions, emotions, and memory. The spinal cord serves as a conduit for signals between the brain and the rest of the body, while peripheral nerves transmit sensory and motor information. The nervous system's efficiency is crucial for overall well-being, as any impairment can affect movement, sensation, and cognitive abilities.

The endocrine system, a network of glands that produce hormones, regulates various bodily functions, including growth, metabolism, and reproduction. Hormones act as chemical messengers, travelling through the bloodstream to target organs and tissues. Essential glands include the pituitary, thyroid, adrenal, and pancreas. The endocrine system's balance is vital for maintaining homeostasis, and any disruption can lead to conditions such as diabetes, thyroid disorders, or hormonal imbalances.

The immune system, the body's defence mechanism, protects against pathogens and foreign invaders. It comprises various cells, tissues, and organs, including white blood cells, lymph nodes, and the spleen. The immune system identifies and neutralizes harmful agents, preventing infections and diseases. A robust immune system is essential for overall health, as a weakened immune response can lead to increased susceptibility to illnesses.

The musculoskeletal system, consisting of bones, muscles, and connective tissues, provides structural support and enables movement. Bones act as the body's framework, while muscles generate force and facilitate motion. Connective tissues, such as tendons and ligaments, connect muscles to bones, bones to bones and stabilize joints. The musculoskeletal system's integrity is crucial for mobility, strength, and overall physical function.

The body's protective barrier is the integumentary system, including the skin, hair, and nails. The skin, the largest organ, shields against environmental hazards, regulates temperature and prevents water loss. Hair and nails provide additional protection and have sensory functions. The integumentary system's health is vital for overall well-being, as it plays a crucial role in protecting against infections and maintaining homeostasis.

The urinary system, responsible for filtering and eliminating waste products from the blood, includes the kidneys, ureters, bladder, and urethra. The kidneys, the primary organs, filter blood to produce urine, which is then transported to the bladder for storage and eventual excretion. The urinary system's efficiency is crucial for maintaining fluid and electrolyte balance and removing toxins from the body.

The reproductive system, essential for producing offspring, includes the male and female reproductive organs. In males, the testes produce sperm, while in females, the ovaries produce eggs. The reproductive system's health is vital for fertility and overall reproductive function.

Each body system is interconnected, and their harmonious function is essential for maintaining health and well-being. Disruptions in one system can have cascading effects on others, highlighting the importance of a holistic approach to health care. By understanding the roles and interactions of these systems, individuals can make informed decisions about their health and well-being, fostering a deeper appreciation for the intricate machinery that sustains life.

The lymphatic system, often overlooked, plays a crucial role in maintaining fluid balance and supporting the immune system. It comprises a network of lymphatic vessels, lymph nodes, and lymphoid organs such as the spleen and thymus. Lymph, a clear fluid, circulates through this network, collecting excess fluid from tissues and returning it to the bloodstream. Lymph nodes filter out harmful substances, while lymphocytes (a type of white blood cell) help defend against infections. The lymphatic system's proper function prevents oedema, supports immune responses, and maintains overall fluid balance.

The sensory systems, including vision, hearing, taste, smell, and touch, allow us to perceive and interact with our environment. Each sensory system is specialized to detect specific stimuli and transmit information to the brain for processing. The eyes, equipped with photoreceptors, detect light and enable vision. With their intricate structures, the ears detect sound waves and facilitate hearing and balance. Taste buds on the tongue detect flavours, while olfactory receptors in the nose detect odours. The skin detects touch, pressure, temperature, and pain with its various receptors. These sensory systems enrich our experiences and enable us to navigate the world effectively.

The body's regulatory mechanisms, such as homeostasis, ensure that internal conditions remain stable despite external changes. Homeostasis involves feedback loops regulating temperature, pH, glucose levels, and other vital parameters. For example, the hypothalamus in the brain acts as a thermostat, regulating body temperature through mechanisms such as sweating and shivering. The pancreas regulates blood glucose levels by releasing insulin and glucagon. These regulatory mechanisms are essential for optimal cellular function and overall health conditions.

The body's repair and regeneration processes are vital for healing and recovery. When tissues are damaged, the body initiates a complex series of events to repair the damage and restore function. This process involves inflammation, cell proliferation, and tissue remodelling. Stem cells, with their ability to differentiate into various cell types, play a crucial role in regeneration. The body's capacity for repair and regeneration is remarkable, but it can be influenced by factors such as age, nutrition, and overall health.

The body's adaptability and resilience are also noteworthy. The ability to adapt to changing conditions, whether through acclimatization to different environments or physiological adjustments to stress, is a testament to the body's dynamic nature. For example, the cardiovascular system can adapt to increased physical activity by improving cardiac output and oxygen delivery. The musculoskeletal system can strengthen in response to resistance training. This adaptability is essential for survival and thriving in diverse conditions.

Understanding the body's systems and interactions provides valuable health and disease insights. It underscores the importance of a holistic approach to health care, considering the interconnectedness of various systems. By nurturing each system through proper nutrition, regular exercise, adequate rest, and preventive care, individuals can support their body's optimal function and enhance their quality of life.

In medical science, technological advancements and research continue to deepen our understanding of the human body. Innovations such as imaging techniques, genetic analysis, and regenerative medicine hold promise for diagnosing, treating, and preventing diseases more effectively. These advancements highlight the importance of ongoing research and the potential for discoveries to improve health outcomes.

The human body, with its intricate systems and remarkable capabilities, is a testament to the complexity and beauty of life. Each system, from the circulatory to the sensory, plays a vital role in sustaining life and enabling us to experience the world. We can enhance our well-being and enjoy a healthier, more fulfilling life by appreciating and caring for our bodies.

Diseases

Diseases have always been a significant part of human existence, shaping history and influencing the development of societies. From ancient plagues to modern pandemics, the impact of diseases on human life is profound and multifaceted. Understanding diseases' nature, causes, and effects on the body is crucial for developing effective treatments and preventive measures. This chapter delves into the complexities of diseases exploring their origins, manifestations, and ongoing efforts to combat them.

Diseases can be broadly categorized into infectious and non-infectious types. Infectious diseases are caused by pathogens such as bacteria, viruses, fungi, and parasites. These pathogens can spread from person to person through contaminated food, water, body fluids, body secretions or via vectors like mosquitoes. Examples of infectious diseases include influenza, tuberculosis, malaria, and HIV/AIDS. On the other hand non infectious diseases often result from genetic, environmental, or lifestyle factors. Common non-infectious diseases include diabetes, hypertension, cancer, and autoimmune disorders.

The body's response to a disease involves a complex interplay of the immune system, genetic factors, and environmental influences. The immune system is the body's primary defence mechanism against infections. It consists of various cells and proteins that identify and neutralize foreign invaders. When the immune system detects a pathogen, it mounts an immune response to eliminate the threat. This response can involve inflammation, the production of antibodies, and the activation of immune cells. However, the immune system can sometimes malfunction, leading to autoimmune diseases where the body immune systems mistakenly identify different body parts as a foreign object and subsequently attacks its tissues.

Genetic factors also play a significant role in the development of diseases. Certain genetic mutations can predispose individuals to specific conditions. For example, mutations in the BRCA1 and BRCA2 genes increase the risk of breast and ovarian cancer. Similarly, genetic variations can influence how individuals respond to infections and treatments. Understanding the genetic basis of diseases has led to the development of personalized medicine, where treatments are tailored to an individual's genetic makeup.

Environmental factors, including lifestyle choices, exposure to toxins, and socioeconomic conditions, can significantly impact health. Poor diet, lack of physical activity, and smoking are major risk factors for non-infectious diseases like heart disease and diabetes.

Environmental pollutants like air and water pollution can contribute to respiratory and gastrointestinal conditions respectively. Socioeconomic factors, including access to healthcare, education, and living conditions, are crucial in determining health outcomes.

A detailed explanation of diseases requires understanding their mechanisms and manifestations. Infectious diseases often begin with the entry of a pathogen into the body. This can occur through various routes, such as inhalation, ingestion, or direct contact with infected surfaces. Once inside the body, the pathogen multiplies and spreads, causing symptoms ranging from mild to severe. The severity of an infection depends on factors such as the virulence of the pathogen, innoculum dose, the individual's immune response, and the presence of underlying health conditions.

On the other hand, non-infectious diseases often develop over time and may not have a single identifiable cause. For example, cardiovascular diseases result from a combination of genetic predisposition, lifestyle factors, and environmental influences. The buildup of plaque in the arteries, known as atherosclerosis, can lead to heart attacks and strokes. Similarly, cancer can arise from genetic mutations that cause uncontrolled cell growth. These mutations can be inherited or acquired through exposure to carcinogens like tobacco smoke and radiation.

The body's response to disease involves various physiological processes. In the case of infections, the immune system's response can lead to symptoms such as fever, fatigue, and inflammation. These symptoms are part of the body's effort to eliminate the pathogen and repair damaged tissues. In chronic conditions like diabetes, the body's inability to regulate blood sugar levels can lead to complications such as nerve damage, kidney disease, and cardiovascular problems. Understanding these physiological processes is essential for developing effective treatments and managing symptoms.

A comprehensive review of diseases reveals the importance of prevention, early detection, and treatment. Vaccination is a crucial preventive measure for infectious diseases, providing immunity and reducing the spread of pathogens. Public health initiatives, such as promoting healthy lifestyles and reducing exposure to environmental toxins, can also play a vital role in preventing certain diseases.

Early detection of diseases can significantly improve outcomes by allowing for timely intervention. Screening programs for conditions like cancer and cardiovascular diseases can identify individuals at risk and enable early treatment.

Treating diseases involves a combination of medical interventions, lifestyle changes, and supportive care. For infectious diseases, antibiotics, antivirals, and antifungals are commonly used to eliminate pathogens. However, the emergence of antibiotic-resistant bacteria poses a significant challenge to treatment. Non-infectious diseases often require long-term management through medications, lifestyle modifications, and regular monitoring. For example, diabetes mellitus management involves blood sugar monitoring, oral hypoglycemic drugs or insulin therapy, dietary changes and lifestyle modifications. Cancer treatment may include surgery, chemotherapy, radiation, and targeted therapies.

Supportive care is essential for improving the quality of life for individuals with chronic conditions. This can include pain management, physical therapy, and psychological support. Chronic pain, for instance, can be debilitating and affect daily functioning. Pain management strategies like medications, physical therapy, and alternative therapies like acupuncture can help alleviate discomfort and improve mobility. Physical therapy is crucial in rehabilitation, assisting individuals to regain strength, flexibility, and function after injury or surgery. Psychological support, including counselling and support groups, can provide emotional relief and coping strategies for individuals dealing with chronic illnesses.

The role of research and innovation in combating diseases cannot be overstated. Scientific advancements have led to new diagnostic tools, treatments, and preventive measures. For example, molecular diagnostics has revolutionized the detection of diseases at the genetic level, enabling early intervention and personalized treatment plans.

Developing targeted therapies, specifically targeting cancer cells without harming healthy tissues, has improved outcomes for many cancer patients. Additionally, the rapid development of vaccines, such as those for COVID-19, showcases the potential of scientific research in addressing global health challenges.

Public health policies and initiatives are critical in managing and preventing diseases on a population level. Governments and health organizations implement vaccination programs, health education campaigns, and disease surveillance systems to monitor and control the spread of infectious diseases. Policies promoting healthy lifestyles, such as anti-smoking laws and initiatives to reduce sugar consumption, aim to curb the prevalence of non-infectious diseases. Access to healthcare services, including preventive care and treatment, is essential for improving health outcomes and reducing health disparities.

The global nature of diseases necessitates international collaboration and cooperation. Infectious diseases, in particular, do not recognize borders and can spread rapidly across countries and continents. Organizations like the World Health Organization (WHO) are pivotal in coordinating global responses to health emergencies, providing guidelines, and supporting countries in strengthening their healthcare systems. Collaborative research efforts, such as those in developing vaccines and treatments for emerging infectious diseases, highlight the importance of sharing knowledge and resources to combat health threats.

Diseases' profound social and economic impact is affecting individuals, families, communities, and nations. Chronic diseases can lead to significant healthcare costs, loss of productivity, and reduced quality of life. Infectious disease outbreaks can disrupt economies, strain healthcare systems, and cause widespread fear and uncertainty. Addressing the social determinants of health, such as education, income, and living conditions, is essential for reducing the burden of diseases and improving overall health and well-being.

The future of disease management and prevention lies in a multifaceted approach that combines scientific innovation, public health initiatives, and individual responsibility. Technological advances, such as artificial intelligence and big data analytics, promise to improve disease prediction, diagnosis, and treatment. Personalized medicine, which tailors treatments to an individual's genetic profile, is set to revolutionize healthcare by providing more effective and targeted therapies. Public health efforts must continue to focus on education, prevention, and equitable access to healthcare services.

Individual responsibility also plays a crucial role in disease prevention and management. Adopting healthy lifestyle choices, such as maintaining a balanced diet, engaging in regular physical activity, and avoiding harmful behaviours like smoking, can significantly reduce the risk of developing chronic diseases. Staying informed about vaccinations, practising good hygiene, and seeking timely medical care are essential for preventing and managing infectious diseases. Empowering individuals with knowledge and resources to take control of their health is a critical component of a comprehensive approach to disease prevention.

In conclusion, the intricate interplay of biological, genetic, environmental, and social factors shapes the landscape of diseases and conditions. Understanding these complexities is essential for developing effective strategies to combat health challenges. Through scientific research, public health initiatives, and individual efforts, significant progress can be made in preventing, managing, and ultimately overcoming diseases. The journey towards better health is a collective endeavour, requiring collaboration, innovation, and a commitment to improving the well-being of all individuals.

Diagnostic and Procedural Terminology

Diagnostic and procedural terminology forms the backbone of medical communication, ensuring clarity and precision in the diagnosis and treatment of patients. This specialized language allows healthcare professionals to accurately describe conditions, procedures, and outcomes, facilitating effective collaboration and patient care. Understanding this terminology is crucial for anyone entering the medical field, as it underpins the entire healthcare process, from initial diagnosis to treatment and follow-up care.

Medical terminology is a complex system of words and phrases derived from Latin and Greek roots, prefixes, and suffixes. These terms are designed to be descriptive and specific, providing detailed information about the patient's condition and the procedures performed. For example, the term "myocardial infarction" precisely describes a heart attack, indicating damage to the heart muscle due to a lack of blood supply. Similarly, "appendectomy" clearly denotes the surgical removal of the appendix. Mastery of this language is essential for healthcare professionals to communicate effectively and avoid misunderstandings that could compromise patient safety.

The importance of diagnostic and procedural terminology extends beyond communication among healthcare providers. It also plays a critical role in medical documentation, billing, and coding. Accurate documentation ensures that patient records are complete and up-to-date, vital for ongoing care and legal purposes. In billing and coding, specific terminology is used to classify diagnoses and procedures, enabling healthcare providers to receive appropriate reimbursement from insurance companies. This system, known as the International Classification of Diseases (ICD) and Current Procedural Terminology (CPT), standardizes medical language across the industry, ensuring consistency and accuracy.

A detailed explanation of diagnostic and procedural terminology involves understanding the structure and components of medical terms. Most medical terms consist of a root word, a prefix, and a suffix. The root word typically indicates the body part or system involved, while the prefix and suffix modify the meaning to provide additional detail. For example, in the term "hypertension," "hyper-" is the prefix meaning "excessive," and "tension" is the root word referring to pressure. Together, they describe a condition of abnormally high blood pressure.

Prefixes and suffixes are essential in medical terminology, as they can significantly alter the meaning of the root word. Common prefixes include "hypo-" (under or below), "brady-" (slow), and "tachy-" (fast). Suffixes often indicate the type of condition or procedure, such as "-itis" (inflammation), "-ectomy" (surgical removal), and "-scope" (visual examination). By combining these elements, healthcare professionals can create precise terms that convey complex medical concepts succinctly.

In addition to understanding the structure of medical terms, it is essential to recognize the various categories of diagnostic and procedural terminology. Diagnostic terms describe conditions, diseases, and symptoms, while procedural terms refer to the methods and techniques used to diagnose and treat these conditions. For example, "pneumonia" is a diagnostic term indicating an infection of the lung parenchyma, while "thoracentesis" is a procedural term describing fluid removal from the chest cavity. Familiarity with these categories helps healthcare professionals accurately describe and document patient care.

A comprehensive review of diagnostic and procedural terminology reveals its critical role in various aspects of healthcare. One key area is patient assessment, where accurate terminology enables healthcare providers to document findings and communicate them effectively to other team members. For instance, during a physical examination, a physician might note "cyanosis" (bluish discolouration of the skin due to lack of oxygen) and "tachypnea" (rapid breathing). These terms clearly and concisely describe the patient's condition, guiding further diagnostic testing and treatment.

In diagnostic testing, precise terminology is essential for interpreting and communicating results. Radiologists, for example, use specific terms to describe findings on imaging studies, such as "pulmonary nodule" (a small, round growth in the lung) or "fracture" (a break in the bone). These terms help other healthcare providers understand the patient's condition and determine the appropriate action. Similarly, laboratory results are often reported using standardized terminology, such as "hyperglycemia" (high blood sugar) or "leukocytosis" (elevated white blood cell count), ensuring consistency and clarity in patient care.

Procedural terminology is equally vital in the context of surgical and therapeutic interventions. Surgeons and other healthcare providers use specific terms to describe the procedures they perform, such as "laparotomy" (a surgical incision into the abdominal cavity) or "angioplasty" (a procedure to open narrowed or blocked blood vessels). These terms provide a clear and detailed description of the intervention, facilitating communication among the surgical team and ensuring accurate documentation in the patient's medical record.

Diagnostic and procedural terminology is used to classify and code diagnoses and procedures for reimbursement purposes in medical billing and coding. The ICD and CPT systems provide a standardized language that enables healthcare providers to document and bill for their services accurately. For example, the ICD code "E11.9" corresponds to "Type 2 diabetes mellitus without complications." In contrast, the CPT code "99213" represents an office or other outpatient visit to evaluate and manage an established patient. These codes ensure that healthcare providers are compensated appropriately for their services and that insurance companies understand the care provided.

The precision of diagnostic and procedural terminology also plays a vital role in research and public health. Accurate and consistent medical terms allow researchers to collect and analyze data effectively, leading to a better understanding of diseases, treatment outcomes, and healthcare trends. For instance, epidemiologists rely on standardized terminology to track the incidence and prevalence of conditions like "influenza" or "hypertension," enabling them to identify patterns and develop strategies to address public health concerns.

In medical education, mastering diagnostic and procedural terminology is a fundamental component of training for healthcare professionals. Medical students, nurses, and other healthcare trainees spend significant time learning this specialized language to ensure they can communicate effectively and provide high-quality care. This education often includes studying the etymology of medical terms, practising their use in clinical scenarios, and applying them in written and verbal communication.

The evolution of medical terminology reflects advances in medical science and technology. As new diseases are discovered and treatments are developed, the language of medicine continues to expand and adapt. For example, the emergence of COVID-19 introduced terms like "SARS-CoV-2" (the virus causing the disease). Staying current with these changes is essential for healthcare professionals to maintain their expertise and provide the best care.

Diagnostic and procedural terminology in clinical practice extends to patient education and communication. Healthcare providers must be able to explain medical terms in a way that patients can understand, ensuring they are informed about their conditions and treatment options. This involves translating complex medical language into plain language while conveying the necessary information. For example, a physician might explain "hypertension" to a patient as "high blood pressure" and describe "angioplasty" as "a procedure to open up blocked blood vessels."

The impact of diagnostic and procedural terminology on patient safety cannot be overstated. Clear and accurate communication reduces the risk of errors and ensures that all healthcare team members are on the same page. For instance, using precise terms to describe a patient's allergies, such as "penicillin allergy," helps prevent adverse reactions and ensures appropriate medication choices. Similarly, accurate documentation of procedures, such as "laparoscopic cholecystectomy" (minimally invasive gallbladder removal), ensures that future healthcare providers understand the patient's surgical history clearly.

Diagnostic and procedural terminology facilitates collaboration among various healthcare professionals in interdisciplinary care. For example, a cardiologist, pulmonologist, and primary care physician might all be involved in the care of a patient with "congestive heart failure" and "chronic obstructive pulmonary disease" (COPD). Standardized terminology ensures that each provider understands patients' conditions and treatments, enabling coordinated and effective care.

The role of diagnostic and procedural terminology in legal and ethical aspects of healthcare is also significant. Accurate and thorough documentation using standardized terms is essential for legal compliance and protecting healthcare providers in case of malpractice claims. It ensures that patient records are complete and can be used as evidence. Additionally, clear communication of diagnoses and procedures supports informed consent, ensuring patients understand their treatment options' risks and benefits.

In summary, diagnostic and procedural terminology is a cornerstone of medical practice, underpinning effective communication, accurate documentation, and high-quality patient care. Mastery of this specialized language is essential for healthcare professionals to navigate the complexities of the medical field and provide the best possible outcomes for their patients. As medical science continues to evolve, so will the language of medicine, reflecting discoveries and advancements in patient care.

Practical Application Scenarios

Imagine stepping into a bustling emergency room, the air thick with urgency and the hum of activity. Doctors and nurses move swiftly, their actions precise and coordinated. Amidst the controlled chaos, a young intern stands at the edge, observing and absorbing every detail. This scene is a vivid example of practical application scenarios in the medical field, where theoretical knowledge meets real-world challenges. Armed with years of study, the intern now applies that knowledge to diagnose, treat, and manage patients in a dynamic environment.

Practical application scenarios are the crucible where medical professionals hone their skills, transitioning from textbook learning to hands-on practice. These scenarios encompass various settings, from emergency rooms and operating theaters to outpatient clinics and community health centres. Each environment presents unique challenges and opportunities, requiring healthcare providers to adapt and respond with agility and expertise.

In the emergency room, the pace is relentless. Patients arrive with a spectrum of conditions, from minor injuries to life-threatening emergencies. The ability to quickly assess and prioritize cases is crucial. For instance, a patient presenting with chest pain requires immediate attention to rule out a heart attack. The intern must swiftly gather a history, perform a physical examination, and order appropriate tests, all while communicating effectively with the patient and the healthcare team. This scenario demands medical knowledge, critical thinking, decision-making, and interpersonal skills.

Operating theatres offer a different set of challenges. Here, precision and teamwork are paramount. Surgeons, anesthesiologists, nurses, and technicians work in unison, each playing a vital role in ensuring the procedure's success. The intern, now a surgical resident, assists in the operation, learning to navigate the complexities of human anatomy and surgical techniques. The sterile environment, the beeping of monitors, and the focused concentration of the team create an atmosphere of intense focus. Every movement is deliberate, every action purposeful. The resident learns to anticipate the surgeon's needs, manage unexpected complications, and maintain composure under pressure.

Outpatient clinics provide a more controlled environment, yet they are no less demanding. Here, the focus shifts to long-term patient care and management. The intern, now a primary care physician, builds relationships with patients, guiding them through chronic conditions, preventive care, and health education. Each patient presents a unique story, a blend of medical history, lifestyle, and personal circumstances. The physician must listen attentively, empathize, and tailor treatment plans to meet individual needs. This scenario emphasizes the importance of continuity of care, patient education, and the art of medicine.

Community health centres extend the reach of medical care to underserved populations. Healthcare providers often face resource constraints and diverse patient needs in these settings. The intern, now a community health worker, engages with the community, conducting health screenings, providing education, and addressing social determinants of health. This scenario highlights the broader context of healthcare, where medical practice intersects with public health, social work, and advocacy. The ability to navigate cultural differences, build trust, and address systemic barriers is essential.

The detailed explanation of practical application scenarios delves deeper into the skills and competencies required in each setting. In the emergency room, rapid assessment and triage are critical. The intern must quickly identify life-threatening conditions, such as myocardial infarction, stroke, or sepsis, and initiate appropriate interventions. This involves interpreting diagnostic tests, such as electrocardiograms (ECGs), blood tests, and imaging studies, and making swift decisions based on the findings. Effective communication with the healthcare team and the patient is essential to ensure timely and coordinated care.

In the operating theatre, surgical skills and knowledge of anatomy are paramount. The resident must master techniques such as suturing, tissue dissection, and hemostasis. Understanding the principles of anaesthesia, infection control, and postoperative care is also crucial. The ability to work seamlessly with the surgical team, anticipate the needs of the procedure, and respond to intraoperative complications is developed through hands-on experience and mentorship.

Outpatient clinics require different skills, focusing on patient-centred care and chronic disease management. The primary care physician must be adept at conducting comprehensive assessments, developing individualized care plans, and monitoring progress over time. This involves managing diabetes, hypertension, and asthma and addressing preventive care, mental health, and lifestyle factors. Effective communication, empathy, and cultural competence are essential to build trust and engage patients in their care.

Community health centres emphasize integrating medical care with public health and social services. The community health worker must be skilled in conducting health assessments, providing education, and linking patients to resources such as housing, nutrition, and mental health services. This role is critical to understanding the social determinants of health, advocating for patients, and collaborating with community organizations. The ability to navigate complex systems, build relationships, and address health disparities is developed through community engagement and interdisciplinary collaboration.

A comprehensive review of practical application scenarios reveals the interconnectedness of medical knowledge, technical skills, and interpersonal competencies. Each setting presents unique challenges and opportunities, requiring healthcare providers to adapt and respond with agility and expertise. The dynamic nature of these environments demands continuous learning and adaptation as medical professionals encounter new cases, technologies, and treatment modalities.

In the emergency room, the intern's journey is marked by a series of rapid-fire decisions and high-stakes situations. One moment, they might be stabilizing a trauma patient with multiple injuries and coordinating with surgeons and radiologists to ensure timely interventions. Next, they could be managing a patient in cardiac arrest, performing CPR, administering medications, and using defibrillators to restore a heartbeat. Each scenario tests their ability to remain calm under pressure, think critically, and act decisively.

Operating theatres, with their sterile precision, offer a different rhythm. Here, the resident's growth is measured in millimetres and seconds. They learn to handle surgical instruments with finesse, make incisions with exacting accuracy, and suture wounds with meticulous care. The resident also gains an appreciation for the choreography of the surgical team, where every member's role is crucial. An anesthesiologist monitors the patient's vital signs, a scrub nurse ensures the availability of sterile instruments, and the surgeon leads the procedure with steady hands and a clear mind. The resident's ability to integrate into this team, anticipate needs, and respond to unexpected challenges is honed through repeated practice and reflection.

In outpatient clinics, the focus shifts to building long-term relationships with patients. The primary care physician's role is akin to that of a detective and a counsellor. They must piece together clues from the patient's history, physical examination, and diagnostic tests to arrive at a diagnosis. They also guide lifestyle changes, medication adherence, and preventive measures. The physician's ability to communicate effectively, show empathy, and build trust is paramount. They must navigate the complexities of chronic disease management, addressing health's medical, psychological and social dimensions.

Community health centres present a broader canvas where the interplay of medical care, public health, and social services is evident. The community health worker's role extends beyond the clinic walls into the neighbourhoods and homes of patients. They conduct health education sessions, organize vaccination drives, and advocate for policies that address health disparities. Their work requires a deep understanding of the community's needs, cultural competence, and the ability to build partnerships with local organizations. The community health worker's impact is measured not only in individual patient outcomes but also in the overall health and well-being of the community.

The journey through these practical application scenarios is a testament to medical professionals' resilience, adaptability, and dedication. Each setting offers unique lessons and challenges, shaping the intern into a well-rounded, competent, compassionate healthcare provider. The transition from theoretical knowledge to practical application is a continuous process marked by moments of triumph, learning, and growth. Through these experiences, the intern evolves into a skilled practitioner, ready to navigate the complexities of the medical field and make a meaningful impact on the lives of patients and communities.

Chapter Review with Interactive Exercises

2.1 Prefixes, Suffixes, and Root Words

Understanding the building blocks of medical terminology is crucial for effective communication in the healthcare field. Prefixes, suffixes, and root words form the foundation of medical terms, allowing for precise and clear descriptions of conditions, procedures, and anatomy.

Key Take aways:

Prefixes: are located before the root words and usually indicate location, time, number, or status (e.g., "hyper-" means excessive, "hypo-" means below average).

Suffixes: are located after the root words and often denote procedures, conditions, or diseases (e.g., "-itis" means inflammation, "-ectomy" means surgical removal).

Root Words: The core meaning of the term, often indicating a body part or system (e.g., "cardi-" refers to the heart, "neuro" refers to nerves).

Exercises:

Prefix Identification: Match the following prefixes with their meanings:

Hyper- (excessive)

Hypo- (below average)

Brady- (slow)

Tachy- (fast)

Suffix Application: Create sentences using words with the prefixes listed above. For example, "The patient was diagnosed with hypertension."

Root Word Exploration: Identify the root words in the following terms and explain their meanings:

Cardiomegaly (cardi-: heart, -megaly: enlargement)

Neuropathy (neuro-: nerve, -pathy: disease)

2.2 Body Systems

A comprehensive understanding of body systems is essential for diagnosing and treating diseases. Each system has unique functions and interrelationships with other systems.

Key Takeaways:

Circulatory System: Transports blood, nutrients, gasses, and wastes.

Respiratory System: Facilitates gas exchange, supplying oxygen and removing carbon dioxide.

Digestive System: Breaks down food, absorbs nutrients, and eliminates waste.

Nervous System: Controls and coordinates body activities through electrical signals.

Musculoskeletal System: Provides structure, support, and movement.

System Matching: Match the following body systems with their primary functions:

S/N		
1	Circulatory	transports blood
2	Respiratory	(breaks down food
3	Digestive	controls body activities)
4	Nervous	provides structure
5	Musculoskeletal	gas exchange

System Function Description: Briefly describe how two body systems interact. For example, "The respiratory system supplies oxygen to the circulatory system, which transports it to cells throughout the body."

System Identification: Identify the body system involved in the following scenarios:

Difficulty breathing (Respiratory System)

Broken bone (Musculoskeletal System)

2.3 Diseases

Knowledge of diseases is vital for diagnosis and treatment. Understanding the terminology helps identify symptoms, causes, and treatments.

Key Takeaways:

Infectious Diseases: Caused by pathogens such as bacteria, viruses, fungi, or parasites.

Chronic Conditions: Long-lasting conditions that can be controlled but not cured (e.g., diabetes, hypertension).

Acute Conditions: Sudden onset and short duration (e.g., appendicitis, acute bronchitis).

Exercise

Disease Classification: Classify the following conditions as infectious, chronic, or acute:

Influenza	Infectious
Hypertension	Chronic
Appendicitis	Acute

Symptom Identification: List common symptoms for the following conditions:

Diabetes (increased thirst, frequent urination, fatigue)

Influenza (fever, cough, body aches)

2.4 Diagnostic and Procedural Terminology

Accurate diagnostic and procedural terminology is essential for effective communication in healthcare settings. These terms describe tests, procedures, and interventions used to diagnose and treat diseases.

Key Takeaways:

Diagnostic Terms: Describe tests and procedures for identifying diseases (e.g., MRI, biopsy).

Procedural Terms: Describe surgical and non-surgical interventions (e.g., appendectomy, catheterization).

Exercises:

Term Matching: Match the following diagnostic terms with their descriptions:

MRI (Magnetic Resonance Imaging)

Biopsy (removal of tissue for examination)

ECG (Electrocardiogram)

Procedure Identification: Identify the procedures described in the following scenarios:

Removal of the appendix (Appendectomy)

Insertion of a tube into the bladder (Catheterization)

Procedure Explanation: Write a brief explanation of a standard diagnostic test and its purpose. For example, "An MRI uses magnetic waves to create detailed images of the organs and tissues within the body, helping to diagnose conditions such as tumours, brain disorders, and spinal cord injuries."

2.5 Practical Application Scenarios

Applying medical terminology in real-world scenarios enhances understanding and prepares for practical use in healthcare settings. These scenarios simulate everyday situations healthcare professionals encounter, requiring the application of knowledge from previous chapters.

Key Takeaways:

Scenario-Based Learning: Engages critical thinking and problem-solving skills.

Interdisciplinary Approach: Integrates knowledge from various body systems, diseases, and procedures.

Communication Skills: Emphasizes the importance of clear and accurate communication in healthcare.

Exercises:

Scenario Analysis: Read the following scenario and identify the medical terms used:

A 45-year-old male presents with tachycardia, dyspnea, and cyanosis. The physician orders an ECG and a chest X-ray to diagnose the condition.

Terms: Tachycardia (fast heart rate), Dyspnea (difficulty breathing), Cyanosis (bluish discolouration of the skin), ECG (Electrocardiogram), Chest X-ray.

Case Study: Write a brief case study using medical terminology learned in previous chapters. Include the patient's symptoms, diagnosis, and treatment plan. For example, "A 60-year-old female with a history of hypertension and diabetes presents with chest pain and shortness of breath. An ECG and blood test revealed a myocardial infarction. The patient undergoes an angioplasty to restore blood flow to the heart."

Role-Playing Exercise: Pair up with a classmate and role-play a doctor-patient interaction. Use medical terminology to describe symptoms, diagnosis, and treatment. For example, "Doctor: 'Based on your symptoms of polyuria and polydipsia, I suspect you may have diabetes. We will need to perform a fasting blood glucose test to confirm the diagnosis.'"

Summary

Mastering medical terminology is essential for effective communication and understanding in the healthcare field. One can decipher the meanings and applications of various medical terms by breaking down complex terms into prefixes, suffixes, and root words. Understanding body systems, diseases, and diagnostic procedures further enhances one's ability to apply this knowledge in practical scenarios. Engaging in exercises and real-world applications solidifies this understanding, preparing individuals for successful careers in healthcare.

CHAPTER 3

ICD CODING PRINCIPLES AND PRACTICE

ICD-10-CM Code Structure

The International Classification of Diseases, Tenth Revision, Clinical Modification (ICD-10-CM) is a system healthcare providers use to classify and code all diagnoses, symptoms, and procedures recorded in conjunction with hospital care in the world. Understanding the structure of ICD-10-CM codes is crucial for anyone involved in medical billing, coding, or healthcare administration. These codes are not just random alpha-numeric sequences; they follow a specific structure that conveys detailed information about a patient's condition and the context of their care.

ICD-10-CM codes are composed of three to seven characters. The first character is always a letter, which indicates the general category of the diagnosis. For example, 'A' and 'B' codes are for infectious and parasitic diseases, 'C' is for neoplasms, and 'D' covers certain conditions originating in the perinatal period. The second character is always a number, further narrowing down the category. The third character can be either a letter or a number, providing even more specificity. These first three characters form the category code, the most general diagnosis level.

The fourth through seventh characters provide additional details about the condition. The fourth character often indicates the subcategory, which gives more specific information about the condition. For example, in the code 'E11.9', 'E' stands for endocrine, nutritional, and metabolic diseases, '11' specifies type 2 diabetes mellitus, and '.9' indicates that it is unspecified. The fifth and sixth characters add even more detail, such as the condition's anatomical site or the disease's severity. The seventh character is often used to indicate the episode of care, such as whether the condition is an initial encounter, a subsequent encounter, or a sequela (a condition that is the consequence of a previous disease or injury).

The detailed structure of ICD-10-CM codes allows for a high level of specificity, which is essential for accurate diagnosis and treatment. This specificity also facilitates better data collection and analysis, which can improve patient care and outcomes. For example, by using specific codes, healthcare providers can track the prevalence of certain conditions, identify trends, and allocate resources more effectively. Additionally, accurate coding is essential for billing and reimbursement. Insurance companies use these codes to determine the reimbursement amount for services provided so that incorrect coding can lead to denied claims or reduced payments.

Understanding the structure of ICD-10-CM codes is not just about memorizing sequences of letters and numbers. It requires a deep understanding of medical terminology, anatomy, and the specific guidelines for coding. For example, certain codes have rules about when they can be used. Some codes require additional characters to provide complete information, while others are considered "unspecified" and should only be used when no more specific code is available. Coders must also be aware of the conventions and guidelines set forth by the World Health Organization (WHO) and the Centers for Medicare & Medicaid Services (CMS), which govern the use of ICD-10-CM codes.

The transition from ICD-9-CM to ICD-10-CM in 2015 significantly changed the healthcare industry. ICD-9-CM codes were limited to three to five characters and lacked the specificity needed for modern healthcare. The expanded structure of ICD-10-CM codes allows for more detailed and accurate coding, essential for today's complex healthcare environment. However, this transition also required extensive training and education for healthcare providers and coders. Many organizations invested significant time and resources into training their staff and updating their systems to accommodate the new codes.

Moreover, the detailed structure of ICD-10-CM codes facilitates better data collection and analysis. This can lead to improved public health surveillance and research. For example, by analyzing data from ICD-10-CM codes, researchers can identify patterns and trends in disease prevalence, which can inform public health interventions and policies. Additionally, the specificity of ICD-10-CM codes allows for more accurate tracking of healthcare utilization and outcomes, which can improve the quality of care and reduce costs.

However, the complexity of ICD-10-CM codes can also pose challenges. Coders must have a deep understanding of medical terminology, anatomy, and the specific guidelines for coding. They must also stay up-to-date with changes and updates to the codes, which can be frequent. Additionally, transitioning from ICD-9-CM to ICD-10-CM required extensive training and education for healthcare providers and coders. Many organizations invested significant time and resources into training their staff and updating their systems to accommodate the new codes. Despite these challenges, the benefits of the ICD-10-CM code structure far outweigh the difficulties, providing a more robust framework for documenting and analyzing patient care.

One of the key advantages of the ICD-10-CM system is its ability to capture a higher level of detail about a patient's condition. This granularity is significant in complex cases where multiple factors may influence the diagnosis and treatment plan. For instance, in the case of a patient with diabetes, the ICD-10-CM codes can specify whether the diabetes is type 1 or type 2, whether it is controlled or uncontrolled, and whether there are any associated complications such as diabetic retinopathy or nephropathy. This level of detail is crucial for developing an effective treatment plan and monitoring the patient's progress over time.

Furthermore, the ICD-10-CM codes are designed to be flexible and adaptable, allowing for the addition of new codes as medical knowledge and technology advance. This ensures that the coding system remains relevant and up-to-date, reflecting the latest developments in medical science. For example, new codes can be added to capture emerging diseases, treatments, or clinical practice changes. This adaptability is essential for maintaining the accuracy and usefulness of the coding system in a rapidly evolving healthcare landscape.

The use of ICD-10-CM codes also facilitates better communication and coordination among healthcare providers. Providers can share detailed and accurate information about a patient's condition, treatment plan, and progress using a standardized coding system. This is particularly important when a patient receives care from multiple providers or transitions between different levels of care. For example, a patient discharged from the hospital to a rehabilitation facility can have their condition and treatment plan accurately documented using ICD-10-CM codes, ensuring that the rehabilitation team has all the necessary information to provide appropriate care.

In addition to improving patient care, the ICD-10-CM codes are critical in healthcare administration and management. Accurate coding is essential for billing and reimbursement, as insurance companies use these codes to determine the amount of reimbursement for services provided. Incorrect or incomplete coding can lead to denied claims, delayed payments, or reduced reimbursement, which can have significant financial implications for healthcare providers. By ensuring accurate and detailed coding, providers can maximize their reimbursement and reduce the risk of economic losses.

Moreover, the data collected through ICD-10-CM codes can be used for administrative and management purposes. For example, healthcare organizations can use this data to analyze patient demographics, disease prevalence, and healthcare utilization trends. This information can inform strategic planning, resource allocation, and quality improvement initiatives. The data can also monitor compliance with regulatory requirements and support accreditation and certification processes.

The ICD-10-CM codes also have important implications for public health and research. By providing detailed and standardized information about patient conditions, these codes facilitate collecting and analyzing large-scale health data. This can support epidemiological research, public health surveillance, and the development of evidence-based policies and interventions. For example, researchers can use ICD-10-CM data to study the prevalence and distribution of diseases, identify risk factors, and evaluate the effectiveness of interventions.

Public health agencies can use this data to monitor trends, detect outbreaks, and allocate resources for prevention and control efforts.

In conclusion, the structure of ICD-10-CM codes provides a comprehensive and detailed framework for documenting and analyzing patient conditions. This system enhances the accuracy and specificity of medical coding, improving patient care, facilitating communication and coordination among providers, and supporting a wide range of administrative, management, public health, and research activities. Despite the challenges associated with the transition to ICD-10-CM and the coding system's complexity, its benefits make it an invaluable tool in the modern healthcare landscape.

Coding Conventions and Guidelines

Understanding the intricacies of coding conventions and guidelines is essential for anyone venturing into medical coding. These conventions and guidelines are the backbone of the coding process, ensuring consistency, accuracy, and compliance across the healthcare industry. They provide a standardized approach to translating complex medical information into alpha-numeric codes, which are then used for billing, reporting, and data analysis. Without a firm grasp of these conventions, coders may struggle to accurately represent patient diagnoses and procedures, leading to potential errors, denied claims, and financial losses for healthcare providers. The importance of coding conventions and guidelines cannot be overstated. They are designed to streamline the coding process, reduce ambiguity, and enhance the quality of coded data. These conventions include general rules and instructions that coders must follow when assigning codes. For example, the ICD-10-CM Official Guidelines for Coding and Reporting provide detailed instructions on selecting the most appropriate codes, sequencing them correctly, and applying various coding rules. These guidelines are updated annually to reflect changes in medical practice, emerging diseases, and advancements in healthcare technology. One of the critical aspects of coding conventions is using punctuation and symbols to convey specific meanings. For instance, brackets, parentheses, and colons in the ICD-10-CM code book indicate different types of information. Brackets are used to enclose synonyms, alternative wording, or explanatory phrases. In contrast, parentheses enclose supplementary words that may be present or absent in the diagnostic statement without affecting the code assignment. Colons are used in the Tabular List after an incomplete term requiring one or more modifiers following the colon to make it assignable to a given category. Understanding these symbols and their meanings is crucial for accurate code assignment. Another important aspect of coding conventions is the use of instructional notes. These notes provide additional guidance on how to apply specific codes and include terms such as "includes," "excludes," "code also," and "use additional code." For example, an "includes" note indicates that the code encompasses certain conditions or terms, while an "excludes" note specifies conditions not included in the code and directs the coder to a different code. The "code also" note instructs the coder to assign an additional code to capture the patient's condition entirely, and the "use additional code" note indicates that an extra code is required to provide more detail about the condition. The conventions and guidelines also address the sequencing of codes, which is critical for accurately representing the patient's condition and ensuring proper reimbursement. The principal diagnosis, defined as the condition that is chiefly responsible for the patient's admission to the hospital, must be sequenced first. Secondary diagnoses, which coexist at admission or develop subsequently, should be sequenced according to their clinical significance and impact on patient care. Proper sequencing is essential for accurately reflecting the complexity of the patient's condition and the resources required for their care. In addition to the general coding conventions, there are specific guidelines for coding certain conditions and procedures. For example, the guidelines for coding infectious diseases include instructions on how to code the underlying infection, the manifestation of the illness, and any associated complications. Similarly, the guidelines for coding neoplasms provide detailed instructions on how to code the primary and secondary sites of the tumour, the histological type, and the behaviour of the neoplasm. These guidelines ensure that coders have the information to represent complex medical conditions and procedures accurately. The detailed explanation of coding conventions and guidelines reveals their critical role in the medical coding process.

These conventions and guidelines provide a structured framework for translating complex medical information into standardized codes, ensuring consistency and accuracy across the healthcare industry. They help coders navigate the complexities of medical terminology, anatomy, and disease processes, enabling them to assign the most appropriate codes for each patient encounter. One of the primary benefits of coding conventions and guidelines is their ability to reduce ambiguity and enhance the quality of coded data. By providing clear instructions on how to apply specific codes, these conventions help coders avoid common pitfalls and errors. For example, using instructional notes such as "includes" and "excludes" helps coders understand the scope of each code and avoid assigning incorrect codes. Similarly, the guidelines for sequencing codes ensure that the principal diagnosis and secondary diagnoses are accurately represented, reflecting the complexity of the patient's condition and the resources required for their care. Another essential benefit of coding conventions and guidelines is their role in ensuring compliance with regulatory requirements. Healthcare providers must adhere to specific coding standards and procedures to receive reimbursement from insurance companies and government programs. Failure to comply with these standards can result in denied claims, delayed payments, and financial penalties. By following the coding conventions and guidelines, coders can ensure that their coding practices comply with regulatory requirements, reducing the risk of financial losses for healthcare providers. The conventions and guidelines also play a crucial role in supporting data analysis and research. Accurate and consistent coding is essential for generating reliable data on patient demographics, disease prevalence, and healthcare utilization. This data is used by healthcare organizations, researchers, and public health agencies to monitor trends, evaluate the effectiveness of treatments, and develop public health policies. Without standardized coding conventions and guidelines, the data collected from medical records would be inconsistent and unreliable, hindering efforts to improve healthcare quality and outcomes. Moreover, coding conventions and guidelines facilitate communication among healthcare providers, insurers, and other stakeholders. These parties can efficiently share information about patient diagnoses, treatments, and outcomes using a common standardized code language. This streamlined communication is essential for coordinating care, processing claims, and conducting audits. It also helps to ensure that patients receive appropriate and timely care, as accurate coding provides a clear picture of their medical history and current health status. The role of coding conventions and guidelines extends beyond the immediate benefits of accuracy, compliance, and communication. They also contribute to the professional development of medical coders. Mastery of these conventions is fundamental to a coder's education and training. Coders must stay up-to-date with annual updates to coding guidelines and changes in medical practice, which requires ongoing education and professional development. This continuous learning process helps coders maintain their expertise and adapt to the evolving healthcare landscape. In addition, coding conventions and guidelines support the ethical practice of medical coding. Accurate and honest coding is essential for maintaining the integrity of the healthcare system. By adhering to established conventions and guidelines, coders can ensure they represent patient information truthfully and avoid fraudulent practices. This ethical commitment is crucial for building trust between healthcare providers, patients, and payers. The complexity of medical coding conventions and guidelines can be daunting, but their importance cannot be overstated. They provide the foundation for accurate, consistent, and compliant coding practices, which are essential for the functioning of the healthcare system. By understanding and applying these conventions, coders can contribute to the quality of patient care, healthcare operations' efficiency, and medical research advancement. In medical coding, the devil is truly in the details. Every punctuation mark, instructional note, and sequencing rule ensures that codes accurately reflect patient diagnoses and treatments. Coders must be meticulous in their work, paying close attention to the nuances of coding conventions and guidelines. This attention to detail sets proficient coders apart from those who may struggle with the complexities of the coding process. The journey to mastering coding conventions and guidelines is a continuous one. As medical knowledge expands and healthcare practices evolve, coding guidelines are updated to reflect these changes. Coders must stay informed about these updates and be prepared to adapt their coding practices accordingly. This dynamic nature of medical coding requires a commitment to lifelong learning and professional growth. In conclusion, coding conventions and guidelines are the bedrock of the medical coding profession. They provide the structure and clarity needed to translate medical information into standardized codes accurately.

By adhering to these conventions, coders can ensure their work's accuracy, consistency, and compliance, ultimately contributing to the quality and efficiency of the healthcare system. The importance of these conventions cannot be overstated, as they play a critical role in supporting patient care, healthcare operations, and medical research.

Advanced Coding Scenarios

Advanced coding scenarios present unique challenges and opportunities for medical coders. These scenarios often involve complex medical cases, multiple comorbidities, and intricate treatment plans that require a deep understanding of coding conventions and guidelines. Mastery of advanced coding scenarios is essential for ensuring accurate and comprehensive documentation, supporting patient care, billing accuracy, and compliance with regulatory requirements.

One of the key aspects of advanced coding scenarios is the ability to code for multiple diagnoses and procedures accurately. Patients often present with various health issues that must be documented and coded appropriately. This requires coders to have a thorough understanding of the coding hierarchy and sequencing rules and the ability to interpret clinical documentation accurately. For example, a patient with diabetes may also have hypertension, chronic kidney disease, and peripheral neuropathy. Each condition must be coded accurately, with the primary diagnosis identified and secondary diagnoses sequenced correctly.

Another critical aspect of advanced coding scenarios is the ability to code for complex procedures and treatments. This often involves understanding the nuances of surgical coding, including using modifiers, bundling rules, and global periods. For instance, coding for a complex surgical procedure such as a coronary artery bypass graft (CABG) requires knowledge of the specific codes for each graft and any additional procedures performed during the surgery. Coders must also be aware of postoperative complications and how to code for them accurately.

In addition to coding for multiple diagnoses and complex procedures, advanced coding scenarios often involve coding for rare or unusual conditions. This requires coders to stay up-to-date with the latest medical knowledge and coding guidelines, as well as the ability to conduct research and seek guidance when needed. For example, coding for a rare genetic disorder may require consultation with clinical experts and carefully reviewing the patient's medical history and documentation.

The ability to code accurately in advanced scenarios also requires strong analytical and critical thinking skills. Coders must be able to interpret complex clinical documentation, identify relevant information, and apply coding guidelines appropriately. This often involves making judgment calls and resolving ambiguities in the documentation. For example, if a patient's medical record includes conflicting information about a diagnosis, the coder must use their knowledge and expertise to determine the most accurate code.

Advanced coding scenarios also present opportunities for professional growth and development. By mastering these complex cases, coders can enhance their skills and expertise, making them valuable assets to their organizations. This can lead to career advancement opportunities, such as becoming a coding supervisor, auditor, or educator. Additionally, coders who excel in advanced scenarios may have a chance to specialize in specific areas of coding, such as oncology, cardiology, or orthopaedics.

The importance of accurate coding in advanced scenarios cannot be overstated. Accurate coding ensures that patients receive appropriate care, that healthcare providers are reimbursed correctly, and that data used for research and public health initiatives is reliable. Inaccurate coding can have various negative consequences, including denied claims, compliance issues, and compromised patient care.

Coders must be committed to continuous learning and professional development to excel in advanced coding scenarios. This includes staying current with the latest coding guidelines and updates, participating in ongoing education and training, and seeking opportunities to expand their knowledge and skills. Professional organizations, such as the American Health Information Management Association (AHIMA) and the

American Academy of Professional Coders (AAPC), offer a range of resources and educational opportunities to support coders in their professional development.

In addition to formal education and training, coders can benefit from networking and collaboration with their peers. Sharing knowledge and experiences with other coders can provide valuable insights and support, helping coders navigate complex cases and stay current with industry trends. Online forums, coding conferences, and local coding chapters are all excellent ways to connect with other professionals in the field.

Advanced coding scenarios also require a strong attention to detail and a commitment to accuracy. Coders must be meticulous in their work, carefully reviewing clinical documentation and applying coding guidelines correctly. This attention to detail is essential for ensuring that codes accurately reflect the patient's medical history and treatment, supporting patient care and billing accuracy.

In summary, advanced coding scenarios present unique challenges and opportunities for medical coders. Mastery of these scenarios requires a deep understanding of coding conventions and guidelines, strong analytical and critical thinking skills, and a commitment to continuous learning and professional development. By excelling in advanced coding scenarios, coders can enhance their skills and expertise, support patient care and billing accuracy, and contribute to the overall quality and efficiency of the healthcare system.

ICD-10-PCS (Inpatient Procedures)

ICD-10-PCS, or the International Classification of Diseases, Tenth Revision, Procedure Coding System, is a comprehensive system used to code inpatient procedures in the world. Developed by the Centers for Medicare and Medicaid Services (CMS), it replaced the ICD-9-CM Volume 3 in 2015. This system is essential for healthcare providers, coders, and insurers, ensuring accurate documentation, billing, and analysis of inpatient procedures. Understanding ICD-10-PCS is crucial for anyone in the healthcare industry, as it directly impacts patient care, hospital reimbursement, and healthcare data analytics.

The ICD-10-PCS system is structured to provide high detail and specificity. It consists of seven alpha-numeric characters, each representing a specific aspect of the procedure. The first character identifies the section of the system, such as medical and surgical, obstetrics, or imaging. The second character specifies the body system involved, while the third character indicates the root operation, such as excision, resection, or insertion. The fourth character denotes the body part, the fifth character represents the approach, the sixth character identifies any devices used, and the seventh character provides additional qualifiers.

One of the critical features of ICD-10-PCS is its ability to capture a wide range of procedures with great precision. This level of detail allows for more accurate coding and billing, leading to better data for analysis and research. For example, the system can distinguish between different types of surgical approaches, such as open, percutaneous, or endoscopic, and can specify the exact body part involved in the procedure.

This granularity is essential for tracking patient outcomes, identifying trends in healthcare, and ensuring appropriate reimbursement for services rendered.

Transitioning from ICD-9-CM to ICD-10-PCS was a significant undertaking for the healthcare industry. It required extensive training for coders and healthcare providers and updates to electronic health record (EHR) systems and billing software. However, the benefits of the new system far outweigh the challenges. ICD-10-PCS provides a more comprehensive and accurate representation of inpatient procedures, ultimately leading to improved patient care and more efficient healthcare delivery.

ICD-10-PCS is not just a coding system but a tool that enhances the entire healthcare process. Providing detailed and precise information about procedures enables healthcare providers to make more informed decisions about patient care. For example, a surgeon can use the system to document the exact location and type of procedure performed, which can be critical for postoperative care and follow-up. Similarly, researchers can use the data to identify trends and patterns in healthcare, leading to new insights and improvements in medical practice.

The system also plays a crucial role in hospital reimbursement. Accurate coding is essential for ensuring hospitals receive appropriate service payments. ICD-10-PCS allows for more precise documentation of procedures, which can help prevent billing errors and reduce the risk of audits and penalties. Additionally, the system supports value-based care initiatives by providing the data needed to measure and improve the quality of care.

ICD-10-PCS is a dynamic system that evolves to keep pace with advances in medical technology and practice. New codes are regularly added to reflect emerging procedures and techniques, ensuring the system remains relevant and up-to-date. This ongoing evolution is essential for maintaining the accuracy and utility of the system, as it allows healthcare providers to document and code new procedures as they are developed.

The detailed explanation of ICD-10-PCS reveals its complexity and importance in the healthcare industry. Each of the seven characters in the code provides specific information about the procedure, creating a comprehensive and precise representation of the medical intervention. This level of detail is essential for accurate documentation, billing, and analysis, and it supports a wide range of healthcare activities, from patient care to research and reimbursement.

The first character of the ICD-10-PCS code identifies the section of the system, which can include medical and surgical, obstetrics, imaging, and more. This initial classification sets the stage for the rest of the code, providing a broad category for the procedure. The second character specifies the body system involved, such as the cardiovascular, respiratory, or musculoskeletal systems. This information is crucial for understanding the context of the procedure and its impact on the patient's health.

The third character indicates the root operation, which describes the primary objective of the procedure. Examples of root operations include excision, resection, insertion, and removal. This character provides insight into the nature of the procedure and its intended outcome. The fourth character denotes the body part involved, offering a precise location for the intervention. This level of specificity is essential for accurate documentation and analysis, as it allows healthcare providers to track and compare procedures across different body parts.

The fifth character represents the approach used to perform the procedure, such as open, percutaneous, or endoscopic. This information is critical for understanding the technique and complexity of the procedure, as well as its potential risks and benefits. The sixth character identifies any devices used during the procedure, such as implants, grafts, or prosthetics. This detail is vital for postoperative care and monitoring, as well as for understanding the long-term implications of the procedure. The seventh character provides additional qualifiers that offer further specificity, such as the type of diagnostic imaging used or the specific technique employed.

The granularity of ICD-10-PCS codes allows for a more nuanced understanding of medical procedures. For instance, consider a coronary artery bypass graft (CABG) surgery. The system can differentiate between a single bypass and multiple bypasses, specify whether the procedure was performed using an open or endoscopic approach, and indicate the exact vessels involved. This level of detail is invaluable for clinical documentation, patient care, and research.

The transition to ICD-10-PCS also significantly changed how healthcare data is collected and analyzed. The increased specificity of the codes enables more accurate tracking of patient outcomes and healthcare trends. Researchers can use this data to identify patterns and correlations previously obscured by the limitations of ICD-9-CM. For example, they can study the effectiveness of different surgical techniques, the impact of various devices on patient recovery, and the long-term outcomes of specific procedures.

Moreover, the detailed coding provided by ICD-10-PCS supports quality improvement initiatives. Healthcare organizations can use the data to monitor performance, identify areas for improvement, and implement evidence-based practices. For example, hospitals can track the incidence of postoperative complications, compare their performance to national benchmarks, and develop targeted interventions to reduce adverse events. This focus on quality and safety is essential for delivering high-value care and achieving better patient outcomes.

The implementation of ICD-10-PCS also has significant implications for healthcare reimbursement. Accurate and detailed coding is essential for hospitals and providers receiving appropriate payment. The specificity of ICD-10-PCS codes helps to prevent billing errors and reduces the risk of audits and penalties. Additionally, the system supports value-based payment models by providing the data needed to measure and improve the quality of care. For example, payers can use the data to assess the appropriateness of procedures, monitor adherence to clinical guidelines, and evaluate care outcomes.

The ongoing evolution of ICD-10-PCS is a testament to its adaptability and relevance. As medical technology and practice continue to advance, new codes are added to reflect emerging procedures and techniques. This continuous updating ensures the system remains current and valid for healthcare providers, coders, and researchers. For example, introducing new minimally invasive surgical techniques or advanced imaging modalities necessitates the creation of new codes to capture these innovations accurately.

The complexity and precision of ICD-10-PCS also underscore the importance of proper training and education for healthcare professionals. Coders and providers must be well-versed in the system to ensure accurate documentation and coding. This requires ongoing education and training and access to resources and tools that support precise coding. For example, healthcare organizations may invest in coding software, reference materials, and continuing education programs to support their staff.

In addition to its practical applications, ICD-10-PCS has broader implications for healthcare policy and planning. The detailed data generated by the system can inform policy decisions, guide resource allocation, and support public health initiatives. For example, policymakers can use the data to identify trends in healthcare utilization, assess the impact of new technologies, and develop strategies to address emerging health challenges. Similarly, public health officials can use the data to monitor disease outbreaks, evaluate the effectiveness of interventions, and plan for future healthcare needs.

The adoption of ICD-10-PCS represents a significant milestone in healthcare coding and documentation evolution. Its detailed and precise codes comprehensively represent medical procedures, supporting various activities from patient care to research and reimbursement. The system's ongoing evolution ensures that it remains relevant and valuable in the face of advancing medical technology and practice. By providing accurate and detailed information about procedures, ICD-10-PCS enhances the entire healthcare process, ultimately leading to improved patient care and more efficient healthcare delivery.

Practical Coding Examples

Examining practical examples can significantly enhance understanding of the intricacies of ICD-10-PCS coding. These examples illustrate how the system's structure and specificity are applied in real-world scenarios, providing clarity and insight into the coding process.

Example 1: Laparoscopic Cholecystectomy

A laparoscopic cholecystectomy, a standard procedure for removing the gallbladder, can be coded with remarkable precision using ICD-10-PCS. The code for this procedure is 0FT44ZZ.

Section (0): Medical and Surgical

Body System (F): Hepatobiliary System and Pancreas

Root Operation (T): Resection

Body Part (4): Gallbladder

Approach (4): Percutaneous Endoscopic

Device (Z): No Device

Qualifier (Z): No Qualifier

This code captures the essence of the procedure, specifying that it involves the complete removal of the gallbladder through a minimally invasive, endoscopic approach.

Example 2: Coronary Artery Bypass Graft (CABG)

A coronary artery bypass graft surgery, particularly involving multiple vessels, demonstrates the system's ability to detail complex procedures. Consider a CABG involving the left internal mammary artery (LIMA) to the left anterior descending artery (LAD) and a saphenous vein graft to the right coronary artery (RCA). The codes for these procedures are:

031209W: Bypass of one coronary artery using the LIMA, open approach

02100Z9: Bypass of one coronary artery using the saphenous vein, open approach

Section (0): Medical and Surgical

Body System (3): Heart and Great Vessels

Root Operation (1): Bypass

Body Part (2): Coronary Artery, One Site

Approach (0): Open

Device (9): Autologous Venous Tissue

Qualifier (W): Left Internal Mammary, Coronary Artery

Section (0): Medical and Surgical

Body System (2): Heart and Great Vessels

Root Operation (1): Bypass

Body Part (0): Coronary Artery, One Site

Approach (0): Open

Device (Z): No Device

Qualifier (9): Saphenous Vein

These codes provide:

- A comprehensive description of the procedure.
- Detailing the specific vessels involved.
- The type of grafts used.
- The surgical approach.

Example 3: Total Hip Replacement

A total hip replacement, a procedure to replace a damaged hip joint with a prosthetic implant, is another example of the detailed coding possible with ICD-10-PCS. The code for this procedure is 0SR90JZ.

Section (0): Medical and Surgical

Body System (S): Lower Joints

Root Operation (R): Replacement

Body Part (9): Hip Joint, Right

Approach (0): Open

Device (J): Synthetic Substitute

Qualifier (Z): No Qualifier

This code specifies that the procedure involves the replacement of the right hip joint with a synthetic prosthesis through an open surgical approach.

Example 4: Endoscopic Sinus Surgery

Endoscopic sinus surgery, often performed to treat chronic sinusitis, can be coded precisely. Consider a procedure involving the removal of tissue from the maxillary sinus. The code for this procedure is 0TBB4ZZ.

Section (0): Medical and Surgical

Body System (T): Respiratory System

Root Operation (B): Excision

Body Part (B): Maxillary Sinus, Right

Approach (4): Percutaneous Endoscopic

Device (Z): No Device

Qualifier (Z): No Qualifier

This code captures the specifics of the procedure, indicating that it involves the endoscopic removal of tissue from the right maxillary sinus.

Example 5: Percutaneous Coronary Intervention (PCI)

A percutaneous coronary intervention, such as placing a drug-eluting stent in the left anterior descending artery, is another example of detailed coding. The code for this procedure is 02703DZ.

Section (0): Medical and Surgical

Body System (2): Heart and Great Vessels

Root Operation (7): Dilation

Body Part (0): Coronary Artery, One Site

Approach (3): Percutaneous

Device (3): Drug-eluting Intraluminal Device

Qualifier (Z): No Qualifier

This code provides a detailed description of the procedure, specifying that it involves the dilation of a single coronary artery site using a drug-eluting stent placed percutaneously.

Example 6: Spinal Fusion

Spinal fusion, a procedure to join two or more vertebrae, can be coded precisely. Consider a fusion of the lumbar vertebrae using a posterior approach with a synthetic substitute. The code for this procedure is 0SG00J0.

Section (0): Medical and Surgical

Body System (S): Lower Bones

Root Operation (G): Fusion

Body Part (0): Lumbar Vertebra

Approach (0): Open

Device (J): Synthetic Substitute

Qualifier (0): Posterior Approach, Posterior Column

This code captures the specifics of the procedure, indicating that it involves the fusion of lumbar vertebrae using a synthetic substitute through a posterior approach.

Example 7: Cesarean Section

A cesarean section, a standard procedure for delivering a baby, can be coded with remarkable detail. The code for this procedure is 10D00Z1.

Section (1): Obstetrics

Body System (0): Pregnancy

Root Operation (D): Extraction

Body Part (0): Products of Conception

Approach (0): Open

Device (Z): No Device

Qualifier (1): Low Cervical

This code specifies that the procedure involves the extraction of the products of conception through an open, low cervical approach.

Example 8: Arthroscopic Meniscectomy

An arthroscopic meniscectomy, a procedure to remove a damaged meniscus in the knee, is another example of detailed coding. The code for this procedure is 0SBC4ZZ.

Section (0): Medical and Surgical

Body System (S): Lower Joints

Root Operation (B): Excision

Body Part (C): Knee Joint, Right

Approach (4): Percutaneous Endoscopic

Device (Z): No Device

Qualifier (Z): No Qualifier

This code captures the specifics of the procedure, indicating that it involves the endoscopic removal of part of the right knee joint's meniscus.

Example 9: Carpal Tunnel Release

A carpal tunnel release, a procedure to relieve pressure on the median nerve, can be coded with precision. The code for this procedure is 01N54ZZ.

Section (0): Medical and Surgical

Body System (1): Peripheral Nervous System

Root Operation (N): Release

Body Part (5): Median Nerve, Right

Approach (4): Percutaneous Endoscopic

Device (Z): No Device

Qualifier (Z): No Qualifier

This code specifies that the procedure involves the endoscopic release of the right median nerve.

Example 10: Kidney Transplant

A kidney transplant, a procedure to replace a diseased kidney with a healthy donor kidney, is another example of detailed coding. The code for this procedure is 0TY00Z0.

Section (0): Medical and Surgical

Body System (T): Urinary System

Root Operation (Y): Transplantation

Body Part (0): Kidney, Right

Approach (0): Open

Device (Z): No Device

Qualifier (0): Allogeneic

This code captures the specifics of the procedure, indicating that it involves the transplantation of a right kidney from a donor through an open surgical approach.

These examples illustrate the depth and precision of ICD-10-PCS coding, highlighting its ability to capture the nuances of various medical procedures. By understanding these practical applications, coders can enhance their accuracy and efficiency, ensuring that each procedure is documented with the utmost detail and specificity.

Interactive Coding Exercises

Engaging in interactive coding exercises can significantly enhance your understanding and proficiency in ICD-10-PCS coding. These exercises provide practical, hands-on experience, allowing you to apply theoretical knowledge to real-world scenarios. Below are exercises designed to challenge and refine your coding skills.

Exercise 1: Appendectomy

A 35-year-old patient presents with acute appendicitis and undergoes an open appendectomy. Determine the appropriate ICD-10-PCS code for this procedure.

Section (0): Medical and Surgical

Body System (D): Gastrointestinal System

Root Operation (T): Resection

Body Part (J): Appendix

Approach (0): Open

Device (Z): No Device

Qualifier (Z): No Qualifier

Answer: 0DTJ0ZZ

Exercise 2: Coronary Artery Bypass Graft (CABG)

A patient undergoes a CABG procedure involving a single coronary artery using the left internal mammary artery. Determine the appropriate ICD-10-PCS code for this procedure.

Section (0): Medical and Surgical

Body System (2): Heart and Great Vessels

Root Operation (F): Bypass

Body Part (1): Coronary Artery, One Site

Approach (0): Open

Device (9): Autologous Artery

Qualifier (A): Left Internal Mammary, Open

Answer: 02100Z9

Exercise 3: Total Hip Replacement

A 70-year-old patient undergoes a total hip replacement of the right hip using a cemented prosthesis. Determine the appropriate ICD-10-PCS code for this procedure.

Section (0): Medical and Surgical

Body System (S): Lower Joints

Root Operation (R): Replacement

Body Part (C): Hip Joint, Right

Approach (0): Open

Device (C): Synthetic Substitute, Cemented

Qualifier (Z): No Qualifier

Answer: 0SR90JZ

Exercise 4: Laparoscopic Cholecystectomy

A patient undergoes a laparoscopic cholecystectomy for gallbladder removal. Determine the appropriate ICD-10-PCS code for this procedure.

Section (0): Medical and Surgical

Body System (F): Hepatobiliary System and Pancreas

Root Operation (B): Excision

Body Part (4): Gallbladder

Approach (4): Percutaneous Endoscopic

Device (Z): No Device

Qualifier (Z): No Qualifier

Answer: 0FB44ZZ

Exercise 5: Lumbar Spinal Fusion

A patient undergoes a lumbar spinal fusion using an anterior approach with a synthetic substitute. Determine the appropriate ICD-10-PCS code for this procedure.

Section (0): Medical and Surgical

Body System (S): Lower Bones

Root Operation (G): Fusion

Body Part (0): Lumbar Vertebra

Approach (A): Open

Device (J): Synthetic Substitute

Qualifier (0): Anterior Approach, Anterior Column

Answer: 0SG00AJ

Exercise 6: Carotid Endarterectomy

A patient undergoes a carotid endarterectomy to remove plaque from the right carotid artery. Determine the appropriate ICD-10-PCS code for this procedure.

Section (0): Medical and Surgical

Body System (3): Upper Arteries

Root Operation (A): Extraction

Body Part (B): Carotid Artery, Right

Approach (0): Open

Device (Z): No Device

Qualifier (Z): No Qualifier

Answer: 03AB0ZZ

Exercise 7: Hysterectomy

A 45-year-old patient undergoes a total abdominal hysterectomy. Determine the appropriate ICD-10-PCS code for this procedure.

Section (0): Medical and Surgical

Body System (U): Female Reproductive System

Root Operation (T): Resection

Body Part (A): Uterus

Approach (0): Open

Device (Z): No Device

Qualifier (Z): No Qualifier

Answer: 0UT90ZZ

Exercise 8: Percutaneous Nephrostomy

A patient undergoes a percutaneous nephrostomy to relieve an obstruction in the left kidney. Determine the appropriate ICD-10-PCS code for this procedure.

Section (0): Medical and Surgical

Body System (T): Urinary System

Root Operation (D): Drainage

Body Part (6): Kidney, Left

Approach (3): Percutaneous

Device (7): Drainage Device

Qualifier (Z): No Qualifier

Answer: 0T9637Z

Exercise 9: Thoracoscopic Lobectomy

A patient undergoes a thoracoscopic lobectomy of the right upper lobe of the lung due to a malignant tumor. Determine the appropriate ICD-10-PCS code for this procedure.

Section (0): Medical and Surgical

Body System (B): Respiratory System

Root Operation (T): Resection

Body Part (0): Upper Lobe, Right Lung

Approach (4): Percutaneous Endoscopic

Device (Z): No Device

Qualifier (Z): No Qualifier

Answer: 0BT04ZZ

Exercise 10: Open Reduction and Internal Fixation (ORIF) of Femur

A patient undergoes an ORIF of the left femur due to a fracture. Determine the appropriate ICD-10-PCS code for this procedure.

Section (0): Medical and Surgical

Body System (Q): Lower Bones

Root Operation (Q): Repair

Body Part (G): Femur, Left

Approach (0): Open

Device (J): Internal Fixation Device

Qualifier (Z): No Qualifier

Answer: 0QPG0JZ

Exercise 11: Laparoscopic Gastric Bypass

A patient undergoes a laparoscopic gastric bypass for weight loss. Determine the appropriate ICD-10-PCS code for this procedure.

Section (0): Medical and Surgical

Body System (D): Gastrointestinal System

Root Operation (Y): Bypass

Body Part (6): Stomach

Approach (4): Percutaneous Endoscopic

Device (Z): No Device

Qualifier (Z): No Qualifier

Answer: 0D164ZB

Exercise 12: Endoscopic Sinus Surgery

A patient undergoes endoscopic sinus surgery to remove polyps from the left maxillary sinus. Determine the appropriate ICD-10-PCS code for this procedure.

Section (0): Medical and Surgical

Body System (C): Respiratory System

Root Operation (B): Excision

Body Part (7): Maxillary Sinus, Left

Approach (4): Percutaneous Endoscopic

Device (Z): No Device

Qualifier (Z): No Qualifier

Answer: 0CB74ZZ

Exercise 13: Percutaneous Coronary Intervention (PCI)

A patient undergoes a PCI with drug-eluting stent placement in the left anterior descending coronary artery. Determine the appropriate ICD-10-PCS code for this procedure.

Section (0): Medical and Surgical

Body System (2): Heart and Great Vessels

Root Operation (D): Dilation

Body Part (3): Coronary Artery, One Site

Approach (3): Percutaneous

Device (B): Drug-eluting Intraluminal Device

Qualifier (A): Left Anterior Descending

Answer: 02733DZ

Exercise 14: Total Knee Arthroplasty

A patient undergoes a total knee arthroplasty of the right knee using a cementless prosthesis. Determine the appropriate ICD-10-PCS code for this procedure.

Section (0): Medical and Surgical

Body System (S): Lower Joints

Root Operation (R): Replacement

Body Part (K): Knee Joint, Right

Approach (0): Open

Device (B): Synthetic Substitute, Cementless

Qualifier (Z): No Qualifier

Answer: 0SRB0JZ

Exercise 15: Open Repair of Abdominal Aortic Aneurysm

A patient undergoes an open repair of an abdominal aortic aneurysm with a synthetic graft. Determine the appropriate ICD-10-PCS code for this procedure.

Section (0): Medical and Surgical

Body System (2): Heart and Great Vessels

Root Operation (Q): Repair

Body Part (4): Abdominal Aorta

Approach (0): Open

Device (J): Synthetic Substitute

Qualifier (Z): No Qualifier

Answer: 02Q00JZ

CHAPTER 4

CPT/HCPCS CODING MASTERY

Introduction to the CPT Code Set

The Current Procedural Terminology (CPT) code set is a critical component in the healthcare industry, serving as a standardized system for reporting medical, surgical, and diagnostic procedures and services. It is developed and maintained by the American Medical Association (AMA); the CPT code set is used by healthcare providers, payers, and researchers to ensure uniformity and accuracy in the documentation and billing of medical services. Understanding the CPT code set is essential for anyone involved in healthcare administration, coding, or billing, as it directly impacts reimbursement, compliance, and overall efficiency in healthcare delivery. The CPT code set is divided into three categories, each serving a distinct purpose. Category I codes represent most procedures and services healthcare professionals provide. These codes are organized into six sections: Evaluation and Management, Anesthesia, Surgery, Radiology, Pathology and Laboratory, and Medicine. Each section is subdivided into specific codes describing individual procedures or services. Category II codes are supplemental tracking codes for performance measurement and quality improvement. These codes are not typically used for reimbursement purposes but provide valuable data for assessing the quality of care. Category III codes are temporary for emerging technologies, services, and procedures. These codes are intended to facilitate data collection and assessment of new and experimental procedures before they are assigned permanent Category I codes. Navigating the CPT code set requires a thorough understanding of its structure and guidelines. Each CPT code consists of five characters, which can be numeric or alpha-numeric, depending on the category. The codes are accompanied by detailed descriptions that specify the procedure or service being reported. Accurate coding requires careful attention to these descriptions, as well as adherence to the guidelines provided by the AMA. These guidelines include instructions on code selection, sequencing, and using modifiers, as well as two-digit codes that provide additional information about the procedure or service. Modifiers can indicate factors such as the location of the procedure, the number of times it was performed, or any exceptional circumstances that may affect reimbursement. The importance of accurate CPT coding cannot be overstated. More than incorrect coding can lead to denied claims, delayed payments, and potential legal issues. It can also impact patient care by affecting the accuracy of medical records and the ability to track and analyze healthcare data. To ensure accuracy, healthcare providers and coders must stay up-to-date with the latest changes to the CPT code set, which is updated annually by the AMA. This includes reviewing the annual CPT codebook, attending coding workshops and training sessions, and utilizing online resources and coding tools. One of the critical challenges in CPT coding is keeping up with the constant changes and updates to the code set. Each year, the AMA releases a new edition of the CPT codebook, which includes additions, deletions, and revisions to existing codes. These changes reflect advancements in medical technology, evolving clinical practices, and the need for more precise and comprehensive coding. Staying current with these updates requires ongoing education, training, and access to reliable coding resources. Many healthcare organizations invest in coding software and tools that provide real-time updates and coding assistance, helping to streamline the coding process and reduce the risk of errors. In addition to understanding the structure and guidelines of the CPT code set, it is also essential to be familiar with the various resources and tools available to support accurate coding. The AMA offers a range of resources, including the annual CPT codebook, online coding tools, and educational workshops and webinars. There are also numerous third-party coding resources, such as coding software, reference guides, and online forums, where coders can seek advice and share best practices. Utilizing these resources can help coders stay informed about the latest changes to the CPT code set and improve their coding accuracy and efficiency. Effective communication and collaboration are also essential for accurate CPT coding. Coders must work closely with healthcare providers, billing staff, and other healthcare team members to ensure that all relevant information is captured and accurately reported. This includes reviewing medical records, discussing complex cases, and seeking clarification. Clear and consistent documentation is critical, providing the foundation for accurate coding and billing. Healthcare providers should be encouraged to document procedures and services in detail, using standardized terminology and formats, to facilitate accurate coding and reduce the risk of errors. The CPT code set plays a vital role in the healthcare industry, providing a standardized system for reporting medical procedures and services. Accurate CPT coding is essential for ensuring proper reimbursement, compliance, and quality of care. By understanding the structure and guidelines of the CPT code set, staying current with updates and changes, and utilizing available resources and tools, healthcare providers and coders can improve their coding accuracy and efficiency. Effective communication, collaboration, and clear and consistent documentation are critical factors in accurate CPT coding. As the healthcare industry continues to evolve, the importance of correct and efficient coding will only continue to grow, making it essential for healthcare professionals to stay informed and engaged in the coding process.

Evaluation and Management Services

Evaluation and management services, often abbreviated as E/M services, are a cornerstone of medical practice. These services encompass various activities healthcare providers perform to assess and manage a patient's health. E/M services ensure patients receive appropriate and timely care, from routine check-ups to complex diagnostic evaluations. Understanding the intricacies of these services is essential for both healthcare providers and patients, as it directly impacts the quality of care delivered and received.

E/M services are categorized based on the complexity and nature of the patient encounter. These categories include office visits, hospital visits, consultations, and emergency department services. Each category has specific guidelines and criteria that healthcare providers must follow to document and bill for services rendered accurately. The documentation requirements for E/M services are detailed and precise, as they serve as the basis for determining the level of service provided and the corresponding reimbursement.

Evaluating and managing a patient's health begins with a thorough history and physical examination. The history component involves gathering information about the patient's current symptoms, past medical history, family history, and social history. This information provides a comprehensive overview of the patient's health status and helps identify potential risk factors or underlying conditions. The physical examination involves a systematic assessment of the patient's body systems, including vital signs, inspection, palpation, percussion, and auscultation. The history and physical examination form the foundation of the diagnostic process.

Once the initial evaluation is complete, the healthcare provider formulates a differential diagnosis, a list of potential diseases that could be causing the patient's symptoms. This list is refined through further diagnostic testing, such as laboratory tests, imaging studies, and specialized procedures. The goal is to narrow the possibilities and arrive at a definitive diagnosis. The provider develops a management plan based on the diagnosis, including medications, lifestyle modifications, referrals to specialists, and follow-up appointments.

The complexity of E/M services varies depending on several factors, including the patient's presenting problem, the amount of data reviewed, and the level of decision-making required. For example, a routine office visit for a minor ailment may involve a straightforward evaluation and management process. In contrast, a hospital visit for a critically ill patient may require a more complex and intensive approach. The service level is classified into levels, ranging from Level 1 (minimal complexity) to Level 5 (high complexity). Each level has specific criteria that must be met to justify the corresponding billing code.

Accurate documentation is crucial for E/M services, as it supports the level of service billed and serves as a legal record of the patient's care. The documentation should include a detailed account of the history, physical examination, diagnostic tests, and management plan. It should also reflect the provider's clinical reasoning and decision-making process. Inadequate or incomplete documentation can lead to billing errors, claim denials, and potential legal issues.

The Centers for Medicare & Medicaid Services (CMS) and the American Medical Association (AMA) have established guidelines for documenting and billing E/M services. These guidelines are periodically updated to reflect changes in medical practice and ensure that providers are fairly compensated for their services. Healthcare providers must stay current with these guidelines to avoid compliance issues and optimize reimbursement.

In addition to the technical aspects of E/M services, effective communication between the provider and patient is essential. Building a solid rapport with patients fosters trust and encourages them to share important information about their health. Active listening, empathy, and clear explanations are critical to effective communication. Providers should also involve patients in the decision-making process, discussing the risks and benefits of different treatment options and addressing any concerns or questions they may have.

The role of technology in E/M services has grown significantly in recent years. Electronic health records (EHRs) have become a standard tool for documenting and managing patient information. EHRs streamline documentation, improve accuracy, and facilitate information sharing among healthcare providers. Telemedicine, which involves using digital communication tools to provide remote care, has expanded the scope of E/M services. Telemedicine offers a convenient and accessible option for patients, particularly those in rural or underserved areas.

Despite technology's benefits, challenges are associated with its use in E/M services. Providers must ensure that EHRs are used effectively and that the documentation is thorough and accurate. There is also a need to balance the use of technology with the human aspects of patient care. While EHRs and telemedicine can enhance efficiency, they should not replace the personal interaction and empathy fundamental to the patient-provider relationship.

Evaluation and management services are a critical component of healthcare delivery. They encompass various activities healthcare providers perform to assess and manage a patient's health. These services are categorized based on the complexity and nature of the patient encounter, with specific guidelines and criteria for documentation and billing. Evaluating and managing a patient's health involves a thorough history and physical examination, followed by diagnostic testing and developing a management plan. The complexity of E/M services varies depending on several factors, including the patient's presenting problem and the level of decision-making required. Accurate documentation is essential to support the level of service billed and to serve as a legal record of the patient's care. Effective communication and technology, such as electronic health records and telemedicine, play a significant role in enhancing the delivery of E/M services.

One of the critical aspects of E/M services is the ability to adapt to each patient's unique needs. Healthcare providers must be flexible and responsive, tailoring their approach based on the patient's circumstances. For instance, a patient with multiple chronic conditions may require a more comprehensive evaluation and management plan than a single acute issue. Providers must prioritize and address the most pressing health concerns while considering the patient's well-being.

The importance of continuity of care must be addressed in the context of E/M services. Continuity of care involves maintaining a consistent and ongoing relationship between the patient and their healthcare provider. This relationship fosters trust and allows the provider to understand better the patient's health history, preferences, and goals. Continuity of care is essential for patients with chronic conditions, as it ensures that their care is coordinated and that any changes in their health status are promptly addressed.

Interdisciplinary collaboration is another critical component of effective E/M services. Healthcare providers often work as part of a multidisciplinary team, including specialists, nurses, pharmacists, social workers, and other healthcare professionals. Collaboration among team members ensures that patients receive comprehensive and coordinated care. For example, a patient with diabetes may benefit from the expertise of an endocrinologist, a dietitian, and a diabetes educator in addition to their primary care provider. Effective communication and collaboration among team members are essential to achieving optimal patient outcomes.

The role of patient education in E/M services must be considered. Educating patients about their health conditions, treatment options, and self-care strategies empowers them to manage their health actively. Providers should take the time to explain medical terms and concepts to the patient in an understandable way.

Visual aids, written materials, and digital resources can enhance patient education and reinforce key messages. Encouraging patients to ask questions and express their concerns fosters a collaborative and supportive environment.

Cultural competence is an essential consideration in the delivery of E/M services. Healthcare providers must be aware of and sensitive to the cultural, linguistic, and socioeconomic factors that may influence a patient's health beliefs and behaviours. Providing culturally competent care involves respecting and valuing diversity and adapting care practices to meet each patient's needs. This may include using interpreter services, being mindful of cultural dietary practices, and understanding the impact of social determinants of health.

The financial aspects of E/M services are also a significant consideration for providers and patients. Accurate coding and billing are essential to ensure that providers are fairly compensated. The complexity of the billing process can be challenging, as it requires a thorough understanding of coding guidelines, payer policies, and reimbursement rates. Providers must stay current with coding and billing regulations changes to avoid errors and optimize reimbursement. Understanding patients' insurance coverage and out-of-pocket costs is essential to prevent unexpected expenses and financial strain.

Quality improvement initiatives play a vital role in enhancing the delivery of E/M services. Healthcare organizations often implement quality improvement programs to monitor and improve the quality of care provided. These programs may involve tracking performance metrics, conducting patient satisfaction surveys, and implementing evidence-based practices. Continuous quality improvement efforts help identify areas for improvement and ensure that patients receive high-quality, safe, and effective care.

The future of E/M services is likely shaped by ongoing advancements in medical technology, changes in healthcare policy, and evolving patient needs. Innovations such as artificial intelligence, machine learning, and precision medicine can potentially transform how E/M services are delivered. These technologies can enhance diagnostic accuracy, personalize treatment plans, and improve patient outcomes. Additionally, healthcare policy changes, such as value-based care models, may shift the focus from volume-based to quality-based reimbursement, incentivizing providers to deliver high-quality care.

In summary, evaluation and management services are a fundamental aspect of healthcare delivery, encompassing various activities that healthcare providers perform to assess and manage a patient's health. These services require a thorough understanding of documentation and billing guidelines, effective communication, interdisciplinary collaboration, patient education, cultural competence, and quality improvement. As healthcare evolves, providers must stay current with technological advancements and policy changes to deliver high-quality, patient-centered care.

Anesthesia, Surgery and Radiology

Anesthesia, surgery, and radiology are one of the pillars of modern medicine that work together to diagnose, treat, and manage a wide array of medical conditions. Each field has its unique history, techniques, and advancements, yet they are deeply interconnected in patient care. Understanding the nuances of these disciplines is crucial for anyone entering the medical field, as they form the backbone of many medical procedures and interventions.

Anesthesia, the practice of administering drugs to induce unconsciousness, paralysis and prevent pain during surgery has revolutionized the field of medicine. Before its advent, surgical procedures were excruciatingly painful and often resulted in significant trauma for the patient. The development of anaesthesia allowed for more complex and lengthy surgeries with minimal discomfort. Anesthesiologists, the specialists in this field, are responsible for assessing patients before surgery, administering anaesthesia, and monitoring vital signs throughout the procedure. They must be adept at choosing the appropriate type and dosage of anaesthesia, whether general, regional, or local, to ensure patient safety and comfort.

Surgery, the branch of medicine involving manual and instrumental techniques to treat diseases, injuries, and deformities, has seen remarkable advancements. From the rudimentary procedures of ancient times to the highly sophisticated methods of today, surgery has evolved to become a precise and life-saving discipline. Surgeons must deeply understand human anatomy, pathology, and surgical techniques. They are trained to perform a wide range of procedures, from minimally invasive laparoscopic surgeries to complex open-heart surgeries. The success of a surgical procedure often hinges on the surgeon's skill, the quality of preoperative and postoperative care, and the effective use of anaesthesia.

Radiology, the medical speciality that uses imaging techniques to diagnose and treat diseases, plays a pivotal role in modern healthcare. Radiologists use imaging modalities, such as X-rays, computed tomography (CT) scans, magnetic resonance imaging (MRI), and ultrasound, to visualize the body's internal structures. These images provide critical information that guides the diagnosis and treatment of numerous conditions. Radiologists must interpret these images proficiently and collaborate with other healthcare providers to develop comprehensive treatment plans. The advent of interventional radiology, which involves minimally invasive procedures guided by imaging, has further expanded the scope of this field.

The interplay between anaesthesia, surgery, and radiology is evident in many medical scenarios. For instance, in the case of a patient with a suspected tumor, radiological imaging is often the first step in identifying the location and extent of the tumor. Once the diagnosis is confirmed, the patient may undergo surgery to debulk the mass, with anaesthesia ensuring that the procedure is pain-free. Radiological imaging may guide the surgery and monitor the patient's progress. This multidisciplinary approach ensures patients receive the most accurate diagnosis and effective treatment.

Various techniques and drugs are employed in anaesthesia to achieve the desired effect. General anaesthesia induces a state of unconsciousness and is typically used for major surgeries. Regional anaesthesia, such as spinal or epidural anaesthesia, numbs a specific area of the body and is often used for procedures involving the lower extremities or lower segment of the abdomen. Local anaesthesia, which numbs a small, specific area, is commonly used for minor procedures. Anesthesiologists must carefully assess each patient's medical history, allergies, and current medications to determine the most appropriate anaesthesia plan. They must also be prepared to manage any potential complications, such as allergic reactions or changes in vital signs.

Surgical techniques have advanced significantly with the advent of technology. Minimally invasive surgeries, such as laparoscopic and robotic-assisted surgeries, have become increasingly common. These techniques involve smaller incisions, resulting in less pain, reduced scarring, and faster patient recovery. Surgeons use specialized instruments and cameras to perform these procedures with precision. Robotic-assisted surgery, in particular, allows for more excellent mastery and control, enabling surgeons to perform complex procedures with enhanced accuracy. Despite these advancements, traditional open surgeries remain necessary for specific conditions and require high skill and expertise.

Radiology has also seen remarkable technological advancements. Developing high-resolution imaging techniques like MRI and CT scans has revolutionized the field. These modalities provide detailed images of the body's internal structures, allowing for more accurate diagnoses. MRI, which uses magnetic fields is beneficial for imaging soft tissues, such as the brain, muscles, and ligaments. CT scans, which use X-rays to create cross-sectional images, are valuable for visualizing bones, blood vessels, and internal organs. Ultrasound, which uses sound waves, is commonly used for imaging the abdomen and pelvis, developing a fetus during pregnancy and other body parts. Interventional radiology, which combines imaging with minimally invasive procedures, has expanded the therapeutic capabilities of radiology. Procedures such as angioplasty, stent placement, and tumour ablation can be performed with precision and minimal discomfort for the patient.

Integrating anaesthesia, surgery, and radiology is essential for managing many medical conditions successfully. For example, in the case of a patient with a complex vascular condition, the collaboration between these fields is paramount.

Radiologists may first identify the issue through advanced imaging techniques, pinpointing the exact location and nature of the vascular anomaly. An interventional radiologist might then perform a minimally invasive procedure, such as angioplasty, to open up blocked blood vessels. Throughout this process, anesthesiologists ensure the patient remains comfortable and stable, tailoring anaesthesia to the specific needs of the procedure and the patient's health status.

In trauma cases, the synergy between these disciplines becomes even more critical. A patient arriving at the emergency room with multiple injuries might first undergo a series of radiological scans to assess the extent of internal damage. These images guide the surgical team in prioritizing and planning the necessary interventions. Anesthesiologists are crucial in managing the patient's pain and physiological responses, allowing surgeons to focus on repairing injuries. This coordinated approach can significantly improve outcomes, reducing the risk of complications and enhancing recovery.

The evolution of these fields has also been marked by significant research and innovation. In anaesthesia, developing new drugs and delivery systems continues to improve patient safety and comfort. Techniques such as total intravenous anaesthesia (TIVA) and target-controlled infusion (TCI) allow for more precise control of anaesthesia levels. Research into the genetic and molecular basis of pain and anaesthesia response is paving the way for personalized anaesthesia plans tailored to individual patients.

Surgical advancements are driven by ongoing research into new techniques and technologies. The use of 3D printing to create custom surgical instruments and implants, for example, is revolutionizing the field. Surgeons can now plan and practice complex procedures using 3D-printed patient anatomy models, improving precision and outcomes. The development of regenerative medicine, including stem cell therapy and tissue engineering, holds promise for repairing and replacing damaged tissues and organs, potentially transforming the future of surgery.

Radiology is also at the forefront of technological innovation. Artificial intelligence (AI) and machine learning are integrated into imaging systems to enhance diagnostic accuracy and efficiency. AI algorithms can analyze vast amounts of imaging data, identifying patterns and anomalies that the human eye might miss. This technology is precious in detecting early signs of diseases such as cancer, where early intervention can significantly improve prognosis. Additionally, advancements in imaging techniques, such as functional MRI (fMRI) and positron emission tomography (PET), provide deeper insights into the brain's functioning and other organs, opening new avenues for diagnosis and treatment.

The training and education of professionals in these fields are rigorous and demanding. Anesthesiologists, surgeons, and radiologists undergo extensive education and training, often including years of specialized residency and fellowship programs. Continuous professional development is essential, as these fields constantly evolve with new research and technological advancements. Medical professionals must stay abreast of the latest developments to provide the highest standard of care.

Ethical considerations are also paramount in these disciplines. In anaesthesia, the potential for adverse reactions and complications necessitates a thorough understanding of patient safety and risk management. Surgeons must navigate complex ethical dilemmas, such as deciding when to operate and balancing the risks and benefits of a procedure. Radiologists face ethical challenges related to imaging technology, including radiation exposure issues and the appropriate use of diagnostic tests. Ensuring informed consent and maintaining patient confidentiality are fundamental moral principles that guide practice in all three fields.

The future of anaesthesia, surgery, and radiology is likely to be shaped by ongoing advancements in technology and research. The integration of AI and robotics, the development of personalized medicine, and the exploration of new therapeutic modalities hold promise for further improving patient care. Collaboration between these disciplines will continue to be essential, as the complexity of medical conditions often requires a multidisciplinary approach.

By working together, anesthesiologists, surgeons, and radiologists can provide comprehensive, effective, and compassionate care to patients, enhancing outcomes and advancing the field of medicine.

Medicine, Laboratory and Pathology

Medicine, laboratory, and pathology form the backbone of modern healthcare, intertwining to create a comprehensive system that diagnoses, treats, and monitors diseases. The journey from symptom to diagnosis often begins in a clinical setting, where a physician evaluates a patient's history and physical examination findings. This initial assessment may lead to ordering laboratory tests, which provide critical data about the patient's health status. These disciplines work together to ensure accurate diagnoses and effective treatment plans.

Laboratory medicine encompasses various tests and procedures to analyze bodily fluids, tissues, and cells. Blood tests, for example, can reveal information about a patient's organ function, electrolyte balances, and infections or inflammatory conditions. Urine tests can detect metabolic disorders, kidney disease, and drug abuse. Advanced techniques such as molecular diagnostics and genetic testing have expanded the capabilities of laboratory medicine, allowing for the identification of specific genetic mutations and the detection of infectious agents at the molecular level. These advancements have revolutionized the field, enabling earlier and more precise diagnoses.

Conversely, pathology delves into the structural and functional changes in tissues and organs caused by disease. Pathologists examine tissue samples, often obtained through biopsies or surgical procedures, under a microscope to identify abnormalities. This microscopic examination can reveal the presence of cancerous cells, infections, and other diseases. Pathologists also perform autopsies to determine the cause of death and to study disease processes in detail. Their findings contribute to our understanding of disease mechanisms and inform clinical practice.

Integrating laboratory medicine and pathology into clinical practice is essential for accurate diagnosis and effective treatment. For instance, a patient presenting with fatigue and weight loss symptoms might undergo a series of blood tests to evaluate thyroid function, blood glucose levels, and markers of inflammation. If these tests suggest an abnormality, a biopsy of the affected tissue may be performed, and the sample sent to a pathologist for examination. The pathologist's findings and the laboratory test results guide the physician in developing a treatment plan tailored to the patient's condition.

The role of technology in medicine, labs, and pathology cannot be overstated. Automation and advanced instrumentation have increased the efficiency and accuracy of laboratory tests. High-throughput analyzers can process hundreds of samples simultaneously, reducing turnaround times and enabling rapid diagnosis. Digital pathology involves:

- Digitizing tissue slides.
- Allowing pathologists to analyze images on a computer screen.
- Facilitating remote consultations and second opinions.

These technological advancements have improved the quality of care and expanded access to specialized diagnostic services.

Education and training in laboratory medicine and pathology are rigorous and comprehensive. Medical laboratory scientists and technologists undergo specialized training in analyzing biological specimens and operating complex laboratory equipment. Pathologists complete medical school, followed by residency training in pathology, where they gain expertise in the microscopic examination of tissues and interpreting laboratory results. Continuous professional development is essential, as these fields constantly evolve with new research and technological advancements.

Ethical considerations are paramount in laboratory medicine and pathology. Ensuring the accuracy and reliability of test results is critical, as these results directly impact patient care. Laboratory professionals and pathologists must adhere to strict quality control measures and maintain the highest standards of practice. Informed consent and patient confidentiality are fundamental ethical principles that guide the collection and analysis of biological specimens. Additionally, test results must be interpreted with care and precision, as misinterpretation can lead to incorrect diagnoses and inappropriate treatment.

The future of medicine, labs, and pathology is likely to be shaped by ongoing advancements in technology and research. Integrating artificial intelligence and machine learning into diagnostic processes holds promise for further improving accuracy and efficiency. Personalized medicine, which tailors treatment plans to an individual's genetic make up and disease profile, is becoming increasingly feasible with advancements in molecular diagnostics and genetic testing. Collaboration between laboratory professionals, pathologists, and clinicians will continue to be essential in providing comprehensive and effective patient care.

In clinical practice, the collaboration between laboratory medicine and pathology is evident in managing complex diseases. For example, in oncology, the diagnosis and treatment of cancer rely heavily on integrating laboratory tests and pathological examination. A patient with a suspected malignancy may undergo imaging studies and blood tests to assess tumour markers. A tumour biopsy is performed, and the tissue sample is sent to a pathologist for analysis. The pathologist's report, which includes information about the type and grade of the cancer, guides the oncologist in developing a treatment plan that may consist of surgery, chemotherapy, and radiation therapy. This multidisciplinary approach ensures that patients receive the most appropriate and effective care.

In chronic diseases, laboratory medicine and pathology are indispensable in monitoring disease progression and treatment efficacy. Patients with diabetes, for example, undergo regular blood tests to measure glucose levels and assess kidney function. Pathological examination of kidney biopsies can reveal diabetic nephropathy, a common complication of diabetes. These insights allow healthcare providers to adjust treatment plans and implement preventive measures to mitigate disease progression.

Integrating genomics and personalized medicine into laboratory medicine and pathology is transforming healthcare. Genetic testing can identify individuals at risk for hereditary conditions, enabling early intervention and customized treatment strategies. For instance, patients with a family history of breast cancer may undergo genetic testing for BRCA1 and BRCA2 mutations. If a mutation is detected, the patient can receive tailored surveillance and preventive measures, such as prophylactic surgery or chemoprevention. Pathologists play a crucial role in interpreting genetic test results and correlating them with clinical and pathological findings.

The advent of liquid biopsy is another groundbreaking development in laboratory medicine and pathology. This minimally invasive technique involves analyzing circulating tumour DNA (ctDNA) in a patient's blood to detect cancer. Liquid biopsy offers a non-invasive alternative to traditional tissue biopsies, allowing for real-time tumour dynamics and treatment response monitoring. Pathologists and laboratory professionals collaborate to interpret liquid biopsy results, providing valuable information for personalized cancer therapy.

In the field of haematology, laboratory medicine and pathology are essential in diagnosing and managing blood disorders. Patients with anaemia, for example, undergo a series of blood tests to determine the underlying cause, such as iron deficiency, vitamin B12 deficiency, or bone marrow disorders. Bone marrow biopsies are often performed to evaluate hematopoiesis and identify malignant cells. Pathologists examine bone marrow samples to diagnose leukemia, myelodysplastic syndromes, and multiple myeloma. These findings guide haematologists in developing targeted treatment plans.

The role of laboratory medicine and pathology extends beyond individual patient care to public health and epidemiology. Laboratory surveillance systems monitor the prevalence of infectious diseases, track antibiotic resistance patterns, and detect emerging pathogens. Pathologists contribute to public health by identifying disease outbreaks and providing insights into disease mechanisms. This information is critical for developing public health policies, implementing vaccination programs, and controlling the spread of infectious diseases.

In forensic pathology, laboratory medicine and pathology intersect to determine the cause and manner of death in legal investigations. Forensic pathologists perform autopsies and analyze tissue samples to uncover evidence of trauma, poisoning, or natural disease processes. Toxicology tests, DNA analysis, and histopathological examination are integral to forensic investigations. The findings of forensic pathologists provide crucial evidence in criminal cases, contributing to the pursuit of justice.

The continuous evolution of laboratory medicine and pathology is driven by research and innovation. Advances in molecular biology, immunohistochemistry, and digital pathology are expanding the diagnostic capabilities of these fields. Researchers are exploring novel biomarkers for early disease detection, developing targeted therapies, and investigating the molecular basis of diseases. Collaboration between researchers, laboratory professionals, and pathologists is essential for translating scientific discoveries into clinical practice.

Integrating artificial intelligence (AI) and machine learning into laboratory medicine and pathology holds great promise for the future. AI algorithms can analyze vast amounts of data, identify patterns, and provide diagnostic insights with remarkable accuracy. In pathology, AI-powered image analysis can assist pathologists in detecting subtle abnormalities and quantifying disease markers. These technologies can enhance diagnostic precision, reduce human error, and improve patient outcomes.

In conclusion, the synergy between medicine, labs, and pathology is fundamental to modern healthcare. Laboratory medicine provides critical data for diagnosing and monitoring diseases, while pathology offers insights into the structural and functional changes caused by disease. These disciplines ensure accurate diagnoses, guide treatment decisions and contribute to understanding disease mechanisms. Continuous advancements in technology and research are poised to enhance the capabilities of laboratory medicine and pathology, ultimately improving patient care and public health.

HCPCS Level II Codes

Healthcare Common Procedure Coding System (HCPCS) Level II codes are essential to the medical billing and coding landscape. These alphanumeric codes, established by the Centers for Medicare & Medicaid Services (CMS), identify products, supplies, and services not included in the Current Procedural Terminology (CPT) codes. This includes durable medical equipment (DME), prosthetics, orthotics, supplies (DMEPOS), certain drugs, and other medical services. Understanding HCPCS Level II codes is crucial for healthcare providers, billing professionals, and anyone involved in the medical reimbursement process.

The HCPCS Level II coding system was created to ensure that healthcare providers could accurately report and bill for various medical services and products. Unlike CPT codes, which primarily cover physician services and procedures, HCPCS Level II codes encompass a broader spectrum of healthcare items. These codes are used by Medicare, Medicaid, and other insurers to process claims for items and services that are not covered by CPT codes. The system is updated annually to reflect medical practice, technology, and policy changes, ensuring it remains relevant and comprehensive.

One of the critical features of HCPCS Level II codes is their alphanumeric structure. Each code consists of a single letter followed by four digits. The letter indicates the category of the item or service, while the digits provide a specific identifier. For example, code "E0118" refers to crutches, while code "J3490" is used for unclassified drugs. This structure allows for high specificity, enabling precise identification and billing of a wide range of medical products and services.

HCPCS Level II codes are not limited to billing and reimbursement. These codes also play a vital role in healthcare data collection, analysis, and reporting. HCPCS Level II codes facilitate the aggregation and comparison of healthcare data across different providers, regions, and periods by standardizing how medical products and services are reported. This data can be used to monitor trends, evaluate the effectiveness of treatments, and inform policy decisions. Additionally, accurate coding is essential to comply with regulatory requirements and avoid potential audits and penalties.

Navigating the HCPCS Level II coding system can be challenging, especially for those new to medical billing and coding. However, with the right resources and training, it is possible to master this critical aspect of healthcare administration. Several key steps can help beginners get started with HCPCS Level II codes.

First, it is essential to familiarize yourself with the structure and organization of the HCPCS Level II code set. This includes understanding the different categories of codes, such as those for DMEPOS, drugs, and other medical services. Each category has its own set of guidelines and rules, so it is essential to review these carefully. Additionally, it is helpful to become acquainted with the HCPCS Level II coding manual, which provides detailed descriptions and instructions for each code.

Second, practice is essential for developing proficiency with HCPCS Level II codes. This can involve working through coding exercises, reviewing case studies, and participating in coding workshops or training programs. Many professional organizations, such as the American Academy of Professional Coders (AAPC) and the American Health Information Management Association (AHIMA), offer resources and certification programs for medical coders. These programs can provide valuable hands-on experience and help build confidence in coding skills.

Third, staying up-to-date with changes and updates to the HCPCS Level II code set is crucial. As mentioned, the code set is updated annually to reflect medical practice and policy changes. Subscribing to industry newsletters, attending coding conferences, and participating in continuing education courses can ensure you know the latest developments and best practices in HCPCS Level II coding.

In addition to these steps, developing a solid understanding of the broader context in which HCPCS Level II codes are used is essential. This includes knowledge of medical terminology, anatomy and physiology, and the healthcare reimbursement process. A solid foundation in these areas will enhance your ability to accurately and efficiently code medical products and services.

The practical application of HCPCS Level II codes can be illustrated through a few examples. Consider a patient who requires a wheelchair for mobility. The appropriate HCPCS Level II code for a standard manual wheelchair is "K0001." If the patient needs a more specialized wheelchair, such as one with a reclining back or power assist, different codes would be used to reflect these features. Accurate coding ensures that the healthcare provider is reimbursed appropriately for the specific type of wheelchair provided.

Another example involves the use of HCPCS Level II codes for billing medications. For instance, the code "J1885" is used for an injection of ketorolac tromethamine, a nonsteroidal anti-inflammatory drug (NSAID). When billing for this medication, including the correct code to ensure proper reimbursement is essential. Additionally, some medicines may require multiple codes to account for different dosages or formulations.

In DMEPOS, HCPCS Level II codes are indispensable for accurately billing items such as oxygen equipment, prosthetic limbs, and orthotic devices. For example, the code "E1390" is used for an oxygen concentrator, while "L5856" refers to a microprocessor-controlled prosthetic knee. Each code carries specific guidelines regarding the documentation and criteria required for reimbursement. Understanding these nuances ensures that claims are processed smoothly and that providers receive appropriate compensation for their services and products.

The importance of accurate HCPCS Level II coding extends beyond financial considerations. Proper coding also impacts patient care and outcomes. For instance, incorrect coding can delay the approval and delivery of essential medical equipment, potentially compromising patient health.

Moreover, accurate coding contributes to the integrity of healthcare data used for research, quality improvement initiatives, and policy development. Accurate or consistent coding can skew data, leading to misguided conclusions and decisions.

In the context of compliance, HCPCS Level II codes are subject to scrutiny by regulatory bodies such as CMS and the Office of Inspector General (OIG). These agencies conduct audits to ensure that healthcare providers adhere to coding guidelines and billing regulations. Non-compliance can result in financial penalties, recoupment of payments, and damage to a provider's reputation. Therefore, meticulous attention to detail in HCPCS Level II coding is essential for maintaining compliance and avoiding potential legal and financial repercussions.

To further illustrate the practical application of HCPCS Level II codes, consider the scenario of a patient requiring home health services. The code "G0156" is used for home health aide services. Accurate coding in this context ensures that the home health agency is reimbursed for the specific services rendered, such as assistance with activities of daily living (ADLs) or personal care. Additionally, proper documentation and coding support the continuity of care by providing a clear record of the services offered to the patient.

Another example involves using HCPCS Level II codes for billing diabetic supplies. The code "A4253" is used for blood glucose test strips, a critical component of diabetes management. Accurate coding and billing for these supplies ensure that patients have access to the necessary tools for monitoring their blood sugar levels, thereby supporting effective disease management and reducing the risk of complications.

In the realm of outpatient services, HCPCS Level II codes are used to bill for a variety of procedures and treatments. For instance, the code "G0463" is used for hospital outpatient clinic visits. Accurate coding in this context ensures that the hospital is reimbursed for the specific services provided during the visit, such as consultations, examinations, and minor procedures. This, in turn, supports the financial sustainability of the hospital and its ability to continue providing high-quality care to patients.

The role of technology in HCPCS Level II coding cannot be overstated. Advances in electronic health records (EHR) systems and coding software have streamlined the coding process, reducing the risk of errors and improving efficiency. These tools often include features such as code lookup functions, automated coding suggestions, and real-time updates to coding guidelines. Leveraging technology can enhance the accuracy and efficiency of HCPCS Level II coding, ultimately benefiting both providers and patients.

HCPCS Level II codes are vital to the healthcare billing and coding system. They enable precise identification and billing of a wide range of medical products and services, support data collection and analysis, and ensure compliance with regulatory requirements. Mastering HCPCS Level II coding requires knowledge, practice, and ongoing education. By understanding the structure and organization of the code set, staying up-to-date with changes, and leveraging technology, healthcare professionals can navigate the complexities of HCPCS Level II coding and contribute to the efficient and effective delivery of healthcare services.

Certification Practice Exams

Mastering HCPCS Level II coding is only complete with vigorous practice and assessment. Certification practice exams serve as a critical tool in this process, providing a simulated environment where aspiring coders can test their knowledge, identify areas for improvement, and build confidence. These exams are designed to mirror the format and content of actual certification tests, offering a realistic preview of what candidates can expect.

Certification practice exams typically cover a broad range of topics, reflecting the comprehensive nature of HCPCS Level II coding. Questions may include scenarios involving durable medical equipment (DME), prosthetics, orthotics, supplies (DMEPOS), outpatient services, and procedures. Each question is crafted to challenge the candidate's understanding of coding guidelines, documentation requirements, and billing regulations.

One of the key benefits of certification practice exams is the opportunity for self-assessment. Candidates can gauge their readiness for the certification test by taking these exams. They can identify strengths and weaknesses, allowing them to focus their study efforts on areas that need improvement. For example, a candidate may discover that they are proficient in coding for DME but need help with the nuances of billing for outpatient services. This insight enables targeted study and practice, enhancing the candidate's competency.

Moreover, certification practice exams help candidates become familiar with the test format and time constraints. The ability to manage time effectively is crucial during the actual certification exam, where candidates must answer a large number of questions within a limited time frame. Practice exams provide a valuable opportunity to develop and refine time management skills, ensuring candidates can complete the test efficiently and accurately.

In addition to self-assessment, certification practice exams often include detailed explanations for each question. These explanations provide valuable learning opportunities, helping candidates understand the rationale behind correct answers and learn from their mistakes. For instance, a practice exam question may ask about the appropriate HCPCS Level II code for a specific type of prosthetic limb. The explanation might detail the criteria for selecting the correct code, including documentation requirements and coding guidelines. This level of detail reinforces learning and aids in the retention of complex information.

Another advantage of certification practice exams is the reduction of test anxiety. Taking a high-stakes certification exam can be daunting, even for well-prepared candidates. Practice exams simulate the testing environment, allowing candidates to become accustomed to the experience and build confidence. By repeatedly taking practice exams, candidates can reduce anxiety and approach the certification test calmly and focused.

To maximize the benefits of certification practice exams, candidates should approach them with a strategic mindset. It is essential to simulate the conditions of the actual test as closely as possible. This means setting aside uninterrupted time, adhering to the time limits, and avoiding external resources during the exam. Treating practice exams as profound assessments helps candidates develop the discipline and focus needed for success.

Furthermore, candidates should review their performance on practice exams thoroughly. This involves identifying incorrect answers and understanding why they were wrong. Reviewing explanations and revisiting relevant coding guidelines can help candidates correct misconceptions and reinforce their knowledge. Keeping a performance record on practice exams can also track progress over time, clearly indicating improvement and readiness for the certification test.

Incorporating certification practice exams into a study plan requires balance. While practice exams are valuable, they should be complemented by other study methods, such as reviewing coding manuals, attending training sessions, and participating in study groups. A well-rounded approach ensures comprehensive preparation and a deep understanding of HCPCS Level II coding.

In conclusion, certification practice exams are an indispensable component of the HCPCS Level II coding certification preparation process. They offer a realistic preview of the certification test, facilitate self-assessment, and provide valuable learning opportunities. By approaching practice exams strategically and integrating them into a broader study plan, candidates can enhance their knowledge, build confidence, and increase their chances of success on the certification exam.

CHAPTER 5

MEDICAL BILLING PROCESSES

Patient Registration and Intake

Patient registration and intake form the cornerstone of any healthcare facility's operations. This initial phase sets the tone for the entire patient experience, ensuring that all necessary information is collected accurately and efficiently. The process involves gathering personal details, medical history, insurance information, and consent forms, crucial for providing quality care and maintaining compliance with regulatory requirements. A well-structured registration and intake process streamlines administrative tasks and enhances patient satisfaction by reducing wait times and minimizing errors.

The importance of patient registration and intake cannot be overstated. It serves as the first point of contact between the patient and the healthcare provider, making it essential to create a positive and welcoming environment. Front desk staff play a pivotal role in this process, as they are responsible for greeting patients, verifying information, and addressing any questions or concerns. Their ability to communicate effectively and empathetically can significantly impact the patient's perception of the facility.

In addition to personal and medical information, the registration process often includes collecting demographic data. This information is vital for various purposes, including public health reporting, research, and equitable healthcare access. Accurate demographic data helps identify trends and disparities in healthcare, enabling providers to tailor their services to meet the needs of diverse populations.

Technology has revolutionized patient registration and intake, offering numerous tools and systems to streamline the process. Electronic health records (EHRs) and patient portals allow for the seamless collection and storage of information, reducing the reliance on paper forms and manual data entry. These digital solutions enhance efficiency, improve data accuracy, and facilitate better communication between patients and healthcare providers. Moreover, they enable patients to complete registration forms online before their appointment, further expediting the intake process.

Despite technological advancements, challenges remain in ensuring a smooth registration and intake process. Common issues include incomplete or inaccurate information, language barriers, and patients' reluctance to share sensitive information. Addressing these challenges requires effective communication, cultural competence, and robust data verification procedures. Training staff to handle these situations with sensitivity and professionalism is crucial for maintaining patient trust and ensuring the accuracy of the information collected.

The detailed explanation of patient registration and intake delves into the steps and best practices involved in this critical process. The first step typically involves greeting the patient and verifying their identity. This can be done by asking for a government-issued ID and matching it with the information on file. Ensuring the patient's name, date of birth, and contact information are correct is essential for accurate record-keeping and communication.

Next, the patient is asked to provide their medical history, including any chronic conditions, allergies, medications, and previous surgeries. This information is crucial for the healthcare provider to make informed decisions about the patient's care. It is important to ask open-ended questions and encourage patients to share as much detail as possible. For example, instead of asking, "Do you have any allergies?" a more practical approach would be, "Can you tell me about any allergies you have and how they affect you?"

Insurance information is another critical component of the registration process. Patients are required to provide their insurance card and any relevant policy details. Verifying insurance coverage and understanding the patient's benefits can prevent billing issues and ensure that the patient receives the appropriate care without unexpected costs. Front desk staff should be trained to navigate insurance verification systems and address patient questions about their coverage.

Consent forms are an integral part of the intake process. These forms include consent for treatment, privacy notices, and any other legal documents required by the healthcare facility. It is essential to explain the purpose of each form and ensure that the patient understands what they are signing. Providing clear and concise explanations can help alleviate any concerns and ensure the patient feels comfortable with the process.

A comprehensive review of the patient registration and intake process highlights the importance of accuracy and efficiency in collecting information. One of the key challenges is ensuring that all information is complete and up-to-date. Incomplete or outdated information can lead to errors in patient care, billing issues, and potential legal complications. Implementing robust data verification procedures, such as double-checking information and using electronic verification systems, can help mitigate these risks.

Language barriers can also pose significant challenges during the registration and intake process. Patients who do not speak the primary language of the healthcare facility may struggle to understand forms and communicate their medical history. Providing translation services and multilingual staff can help bridge this gap and ensure all patients receive the necessary care. Additionally, using clear and straight forward language in forms and verbal communication can make the process more accessible to all patients.

Patients' reluctance to share sensitive information is another common issue. Concerns about privacy and confidentiality can lead to incomplete or inaccurate information being provided. Building trust with patients is essential for overcoming this barrier. Front desk staff should be trained to explain the facility's privacy policies and reassure patients that their information will be kept confidential. Creating a welcoming and non-judgmental environment encourages patients to share more openly.

Technology plays a crucial role in enhancing the patient registration and intake process. Electronic health records (EHRs) and patient portals have become indispensable tools in modern healthcare settings. EHRs allow for the seamless integration of patient information across various departments, ensuring healthcare providers access to up-to-date and comprehensive data. This integration improves the quality of care and reduces the likelihood of errors and duplicative tests. On the other hand, patient portals empower patients to take an active role in their healthcare by allowing them to complete registration forms, update their information, and communicate with their providers online.

Digital solutions also enhance the efficiency of the registration and intake process. Automated systems can flag incomplete or inconsistent information, prompting staff to address these issues before they become problematic. Additionally, digital forms can guide patients through the process step-by-step, reducing the likelihood of errors and ensuring that all necessary information is collected. These systems can also streamline the workflow for front desk staff, allowing them to focus on more complex tasks and provide better patient service.

Despite the many benefits of technology, it is essential to recognize that not all patients may be comfortable or familiar with digital tools. Providing alternative options, such as paper forms or in-person assistance, ensures that all patients can complete the registration process regardless of technological proficiency. Training staff to assist patients with digital tools and addressing any technical issues that may arise is also crucial for maintaining a smooth and efficient process.

The role of front desk staff in the registration and intake process cannot be overstated. These individuals are often the first point of contact for patients, and their ability to communicate effectively and empathetically can significantly impact the patient's experience. Training front desk staff in customer service, cultural competence, and data verification procedures is essential for ensuring a positive and efficient registration process. Additionally, providing ongoing training and support can help staff stay up-to-date with the latest tools and best practices.

Effective communication is a critical component of the registration and intake process. Clear and concise explanations of forms, procedures, and policies can help alleviate patient concerns and ensure that they understand what is required of them. Open-ended questions and active listening techniques can encourage patients to share more detailed information about their medical history and concerns. For example, instead of asking, "Do you have any medical conditions?" a more practical approach would be, "Can you tell me about any medical conditions you have and how they affect your daily life?"

Cultural competence is another essential aspect of the registration and intake process. Understanding and respecting patients' diverse backgrounds and needs can help create a more inclusive and welcoming environment. Providing training on cultural competence and offering translation services can help staff communicate more effectively with patients from different cultural backgrounds. Additionally, awareness of cultural differences in communication styles and healthcare beliefs can help staff build trust and rapport with patients.

Data verification is critical in ensuring the accuracy and completeness of the information collected during the registration and intake process. Implementing procedures for double-checking information, such as verifying patient details with a government-issued ID and cross-referencing information with existing records, can help prevent errors and ensure the patient's information is accurate. Additionally, using electronic verification systems can streamline this process and reduce the likelihood of human error.

The patient registration and intake process is a complex and multifaceted task that requires careful attention to detail and effective communication. By leveraging technology, providing comprehensive training for front desk staff, and addressing common challenges such as language barriers and patients' reluctance to share sensitive information, healthcare facilities can create a more efficient and positive experience for patients. Ensuring that all necessary information is collected accurately and efficiently is essential for providing quality care and maintaining compliance with regulatory requirements.

In summary, the patient registration and intake process is a critical component of healthcare operations that sets the foundation for the patient experience. By focusing on accuracy, efficiency, and effective communication, healthcare facilities can enhance patient satisfaction, improve the quality of care, and streamline administrative tasks. Leveraging technology and providing comprehensive training for front desk staff are vital strategies for achieving these goals and ensuring a smooth and efficient registration process.

Charge Capture and Claims Creation

Charge capture and claims creation are pivotal in the healthcare revenue cycle, ensuring services are accurately documented and billed. These processes are essential for maintaining financial stability and compliance within healthcare organizations. Charge capture involves recording the services provided to patients, while claims creation entails compiling this information into a format suitable for submission to insurance companies for reimbursement. Both processes require meticulous attention to detail and a thorough understanding of coding and billing regulations.

The importance of charge capture cannot be overstated. Accurate charge capture ensures that healthcare providers are compensated for their services. This process begins at the point of care, where clinicians document the services and procedures performed. This documentation is then translated into standardized codes, such as Current Procedural Terminology (CPT) codes, which communicate the nature of the services to payers.

Errors in charge capture can lead to significant financial losses, as services may be undercoded, overcoded, or omitted entirely. Therefore, healthcare providers must implement robust charge capture systems and provide ongoing training to staff to ensure accuracy.

Claims creation is the next step in the revenue cycle, where the captured charges are compiled into claims for submission to insurance companies. This process involves verifying patient information, ensuring that the patient's insurance plan covers the services, and applying the appropriate codes and modifiers. Claims must be submitted promptly to avoid delays in reimbursement. Also, claims must comply with payer requirements and regulations to prevent denials and audits. The complexity of claims creation necessitates a thorough understanding of billing guidelines and the ability to navigate various payer systems.

Technology integration has significantly improved charge capture and claims creation efficiency and accuracy. Electronic health records (EHRs) and practice management systems streamline the documentation and coding process, reducing the likelihood of errors. Before submitting claims, these systems can also flag potential issues, such as missing information or incorrect codes. Additionally, automated charge capture tools can extract relevant data from clinical documentation, further enhancing accuracy and efficiency. However, it is essential to recognize that technology is not a panacea; human oversight and expertise are still necessary to ensure the integrity of the process.

Effective charge capture and claims creation require collaboration among various stakeholders within the healthcare organization. Clinicians, coders, billers, and administrative staff must work together to ensure services are accurately documented and billed. Clear communication and defined workflows are essential for preventing errors and capturing all charges. Regular audits and reviews help identify improvement areas and ensure billing regulations compliance. Additionally, providing ongoing education and training to staff can help them stay current with coding and billing guidelines and enhance their proficiency.

The financial health of a healthcare organization is closely tied to the effectiveness of its charge capture and claims creation processes. Accurate and timely charge capture ensures that all services provided are billed, maximizing revenue and reducing the risk of financial losses. Efficient claims creation and submission processes minimize delays in reimbursement and reduce the likelihood of denials. By investing in robust charge capture and claims creation systems and providing ongoing training and support to staff, healthcare organizations can enhance their financial performance and ensure compliance with regulatory requirements.

Charge capture and claims creation are not without their challenges. One common issue is the complexity of coding and billing regulations, which can vary by payer and change frequently. Keeping up with these changes requires continuous education and vigilance. Additionally, discrepancies between clinical documentation and coding can lead to errors and denials. Ensuring that clinicians provide detailed and accurate documentation is essential for accurate charge capture. Another challenge is the potential for human error, which can occur at any process stage. Implementing checks and balances, such as automated tools and regular audits, can help mitigate this risk.

The role of technology in charge capture and claims creation cannot be overlooked. EHRs and practice management systems have revolutionized these processes, making them more efficient and accurate. These systems can automate many aspects of charge capture and claims creation, reducing the burden on staff and minimizing the risk of errors. For example, automated charge capture tools can extract relevant data from clinical documentation and apply the appropriate codes, while practice management systems can streamline the claims submission process. However, it is crucial to recognize that technology is not a substitute for human expertise. Staff must be trained to use these systems effectively and identify and address any issues.

Collaboration and communication are essential to successful charge capture and claims creation. Clinicians, coders, billers, and administrative staff must work together to ensure services are accurately documented and billed. Clear communication and defined workflows can help prevent errors and capture all charges. Regular audits and reviews can help identify areas for improvement and ensure compliance with billing regulations. Additionally, providing ongoing education and training to staff can help them stay current with coding and billing guidelines and enhance their proficiency.

The financial health of a healthcare organization is closely tied to the effectiveness of its charge capture and claims creation processes. Accurate and timely charge capture ensures that all services provided are billed, maximizing revenue and reducing the risk of financial losses. Efficient claims creation and submission processes minimize delays in reimbursement and reduce the likelihood of denials. By investing in robust charge capture and claims creation systems and providing ongoing training and support to staff, healthcare organizations can enhance their financial performance and ensure compliance with regulatory requirements.

One of the most significant challenges in charge capture and claims creation is the ever-evolving landscape of healthcare regulations. Payers frequently update their policies, and new coding guidelines are introduced regularly. This dynamic environment requires healthcare organizations to stay vigilant and adaptable. Regular training sessions and updates for staff are essential to keep everyone informed about the latest changes. Additionally, subscribing to industry newsletters and participating in professional organizations can provide valuable insights and resources to stay current with regulatory developments.

Another critical aspect of charge capture and claims creation is the importance of accurate and detailed clinical documentation. Clinicians play a crucial role in this process, as their documentation is the foundation for coding and billing. Incomplete or vague documentation can lead to coding errors and potential denials. Encouraging clinicians to provide comprehensive and specific documentation can significantly improve charge capture accuracy. Implementing standardized templates and documentation guidelines can also help streamline this process and ensure consistency across the organization.

The role of coders and billers in capturing and claims creation cannot be underestimated. These professionals possess specialized knowledge and skills essential for accurate coding and billing. Investing in their education and professional development can enhance their proficiency and ensure that they stay current with industry standards. Additionally, fostering a collaborative environment where coders and billers can communicate with clinicians and other staff members can help address any discrepancies or issues that may arise during the charge capture and claims creation process.

Technology continues to play a transformative role in charge capture and claims creation. Advanced analytics and artificial intelligence (AI) tools are increasingly used to identify billing data patterns and trends, helping organizations optimize their revenue cycle processes. For example, predictive analytics can identify potential coding errors or discrepancies before submitting claims, reducing the likelihood of denials. AI-powered tools can also assist in automating routine tasks, such as data entry and claims submission, freeing staff to focus on more complex and value-added activities.

Despite technological advancements, human oversight remains essential in charge capture and claims creation. Automated systems can flag potential issues, but it is ultimately up to trained professionals to review and address these concerns. Regular audits and quality assurance checks can help identify gaps or areas for improvement in the process. Additionally, fostering a culture of accountability and continuous improvement can encourage staff to take ownership of their roles and strive for excellence in charge capture and claims creation.

Effective charge capture and claims creation are crucial for financial stability and compliance with regulatory requirements. Healthcare organizations must adhere to strict guidelines and standards to avoid penalties and audits. Implementing robust compliance programs and conducting regular internal audits can help ensure the organization complies with all applicable regulations. Additionally, staying informed about changes in regulatory requirements and proactively addressing any potential issues can help mitigate risks and protect the organization's reputation.

In conclusion, charge capture and claims creation are integral to the healthcare revenue cycle. Accurate and efficient processes in these areas are essential for maximizing revenue, minimizing denials, and ensuring compliance with regulatory requirements. By investing in technology, providing ongoing training and support to staff, and fostering a collaborative and accountable environment, healthcare organizations can enhance their charge capture and claims creation processes and achieve financial success.

Billing Rules and Procedures

Navigating the healthcare industry's labyrinth of billing rules and procedures can be daunting, especially for beginners. The complexity arises from the myriad of regulations, payer-specific guidelines, and the need for meticulous documentation. Understanding these rules is crucial for ensuring timely and accurate reimbursement, maintaining compliance, and avoiding costly denials. This chapter delves into the intricacies of billing rules and procedures, offering practical advice and actionable steps to streamline the process.

Billing in healthcare is governed by a set of rules and procedures designed to standardize the process and ensure compliance with regulatory requirements. Various entities, including federal and state governments, private insurers, and accrediting organizations, establish these rules. Each payer may have its guidelines, making it essential for healthcare providers to stay informed and adaptable. The foundation of effective billing lies in understanding these rules and implementing procedures that align with them.

One of the fundamental aspects of billing is using standardized codes to represent medical services and procedures. The International Classification of Diseases (ICD) and the Current Procedural Terminology (CPT) codes are the most commonly used coding systems. Accurate coding is critical for ensuring that claims are processed correctly and that providers receive appropriate reimbursement. Errors in coding can lead to claim denials, payment delays, and potential audits. Therefore, it is essential for billing staff to be well-versed in these coding systems and to stay updated on any changes or updates.

Another critical component of billing is the submission of claims to payers. This process involves several steps, including verifying patient information, ensuring that the patient's insurance plan covers services, and submitting the claim electronically or via paper. Each payer may have specific requirements for claim submission, such as the claim format, required documentation, and timelines for submission. Adhering to these requirements is crucial for avoiding denials and ensuring timely payment.

In addition to coding and claim submission, billing rules and procedures encompass denials and appeals management. Denials occur when a payer refuses to pay for a service or procedure, often due to errors in coding, lack of documentation, or non-compliance with payer guidelines. Managing denials involves identifying the reason for the denial, correcting any mistakes, and resubmitting the claim. Sometimes, it may be necessary to appeal the denial, providing additional documentation or justification for the service. Effective denial management is essential for maximizing revenue and minimizing financial losses.

The role of technology in billing cannot be overstated. Electronic health records (EHR) systems, practice management software, and billing platforms can streamline the billing process, reduce errors, and improve efficiency. These tools can automate many aspects of billing, such as coding, claim submission, and denial management, freeing up staff to focus on more complex tasks. However, ensuring these systems are correctly configured and regularly updated is essential to comply with current billing rules and procedures.

Training and education are also critical components of effective billing. Billing staff must know coding systems, payer guidelines, and regulatory requirements. Ongoing training and professional development can help staff stay current with changes in the industry and improve their skills. Additionally, fostering a culture of continuous improvement and accountability can encourage staff to take ownership of their roles and strive for excellence in billing.

Billing rules and procedures are not static; they evolve in response to changes in healthcare regulations, payer policies, and industry standards. Staying informed about these changes is essential for maintaining compliance and optimizing revenue. Subscribing to industry newsletters, participating in professional organizations, and attending conferences and workshops can provide valuable insights and resources for staying current with billing rules and procedures.

Effective communication and collaboration among billing staff, clinicians, and other stakeholders are also crucial for successful billing. Clear and consistent communication can help ensure everyone is on the same page and that any issues or discrepancies are promptly addressed. Regular meetings and updates can facilitate this communication and allow staff to share knowledge and best practices.

Understanding and adhering to billing rules and procedures is essential for ensuring accurate and timely reimbursement, maintaining compliance, and avoiding costly denials. By investing in training and education, leveraging technology, and fostering a culture of continuous improvement and collaboration, healthcare providers can streamline their billing processes and achieve financial success.

Payment Adjudication and Denial Management

Payment adjudication and denial management are critical components of the healthcare revenue cycle. These processes ensure healthcare providers receive appropriate reimbursement for services rendered while minimizing financial losses due to denied claims. Payment adjudication involves reviewing and processing payers' claims to determine the reimbursement amount. Denial management, on the other hand, focuses on identifying, addressing, and preventing claim denials. Both processes require a thorough understanding of payer guidelines, coding systems, and regulatory requirements.

The journey of a claim begins with its submission to the payer. Once received, the payer's adjudication system evaluates the claim based on various criteria, including patient eligibility, coverage, medical necessity, and coding accuracy. This evaluation determines whether the claim will be approved, partially paid, or denied. The adjudication process is complex and involves multiple steps, including initial review, automated edits, manual review, and final determination. Each step is designed to ensure that the claim meets the payer's requirements and that the reimbursement is accurate.

Denial management is essential to the revenue cycle, as denied claims can significantly impact a healthcare provider's financial health. Denials can occur for various reasons, including incorrect coding, lack of documentation, non-compliance with payer guidelines, and eligibility issues. Effective denial management involves identifying the root causes of denials, implementing corrective actions, and resubmitting claims for reconsideration. It also requires a proactive approach to prevent future denials by addressing common issues and improving processes.

One of the key strategies for effective denial management is establishing a robust denial tracking system. This system should capture detailed information about each denial, including the reason, the payer's explanation, and any actions to address the issue. By analyzing this data, healthcare providers can identify patterns and trends, allowing them to target specific areas for improvement. For example, additional training for coding staff may be necessary if many denials are due to coding errors.

Another critical aspect of denial management is the appeals process. When a claim is denied, healthcare providers can appeal the decision. The appeals process involves submitting additional documentation or providing a detailed explanation to support the claim.

It is essential to follow the payer's guidelines for appeals, including timelines and required documentation. A well-prepared appeal can increase the likelihood of overturning the denial and securing reimbursement.

Collaboration and communication among billing staff, clinicians, and other stakeholders are crucial for successful denial management. Billing staff must work closely with clinicians to ensure that documentation is complete and accurate. Regular meetings and updates can facilitate this collaboration and provide opportunities for staff to share knowledge and best practices. Additionally, fostering a culture of accountability and continuous improvement can encourage staff to take ownership of their roles and strive for excellence in denial management.

Technology plays a significant role in both payment adjudication and denial management. Electronic health records (EHR) systems, practice management software, and billing platforms can streamline these processes, reduce errors, and improve efficiency. These tools can automate many adjudication and denial management aspects, such as coding, claim submission, and tracking. However, ensuring these systems are correctly configured and regularly updated is vital to comply with current payer guidelines and regulatory requirements.

Training and education are critical components of effective payment adjudication and denial management. Billing staff must know coding systems, payer guidelines, and regulatory requirements. Ongoing training and professional development can help staff stay current with changes in the industry and improve their skills. Also, fostering a continuous improvement and accountability culture can encourage staff to take ownership of their roles and strive for excellence in these processes.

Payment adjudication and denial management are not static; they evolve in response to changes in healthcare regulations, payer policies, and industry standards. Staying informed about these changes is essential for maintaining compliance and optimizing revenue. Subscribing to industry newsletters, participating in professional organizations, and attending conferences and workshops can provide valuable insights and resources for staying current with payment adjudication and denial management.

Effective communication and collaboration among billing staff, clinicians, and other stakeholders are crucial for successful payment adjudication and denial management. Clear and consistent communication can help ensure everyone is on the same page and that any issues or discrepancies are promptly addressed. Regular meetings and updates can facilitate this communication and allow staff to share knowledge and best practices.

Understanding and adhering to payment adjudication and denial management processes is essential for ensuring accurate and timely reimbursement, maintaining compliance, and avoiding costly denials. By investing in training and education, leveraging technology, and fostering a culture of continuous improvement and collaboration, healthcare providers can streamline their payment adjudication and denial management processes and achieve financial success.

Patient Billing and Collections

Patient billing and collections form the backbone of a healthcare provider's financial health. Navigating this complex landscape requires precision, empathy, and efficiency. The process begins when a patient schedules an appointment and continues until the final payment is received. Each step in this journey is crucial, as errors or delays can lead to financial strain for both the provider and the patient. Understanding the intricacies of patient billing and collections is essential for maintaining a sustainable practice and ensuring patient satisfaction.

The billing process starts with accurate patient information. Collecting comprehensive data during the initial registration phase sets the stage for smooth billing operations. This includes personal details, insurance information, and any relevant medical history. Ensuring this information is correct and up-to-date minimizes the risk of claim denials and delays. Front-end staff play a pivotal role in this phase, as their attention to detail can significantly impact the overall efficiency of the billing cycle.

Once the patient visit is complete, the billing department takes over. Coding the services provided accurately is paramount. Medical coders translate the healthcare services into standardized codes, which are then used to generate claims. These claims are submitted to insurance companies for reimbursement. Coding accuracy cannot be overstated; incorrect codes can lead to claim rejections, necessitating time-consuming corrections and resubmissions. Investing in trained coders and regular audits can mitigate these risks.

Insurance verification and pre-authorization are critical steps that often occur before the patient enters the office. Verifying insurance coverage ensures that the services provided will be covered, reducing the likelihood of unexpected out-of-pocket expenses for the patient. Pre-authorization, conversely, involves obtaining approval from the insurance company for specific procedures or treatments. This step is crucial for high-cost services, as it guarantees that the provider will be reimbursed.

Patient billing continues after insurance claims. Once the insurance company processes the claim, any remaining balance is billed to the patient. This is where clear communication becomes essential. Sending detailed, easy-to-understand statements helps patients comprehend their financial responsibilities. Including a breakdown of charges, insurance payments, and any adjustments can prevent confusion and disputes. Multiple payment options, such as online payments, payment plans, and credit card payments, can facilitate timely collections.

Collections can be a delicate aspect of patient billing. While recovering outstanding balances is essential, it's equally crucial to approach collections with empathy. Patients may face financial hardships, and a compassionate approach can make a significant difference. Establishing and communicating a clear collections policy to patients upfront can set expectations and reduce misunderstandings. For overdue accounts, gentle reminders and follow-up calls can be effective. Sometimes, partnering with a collections agency may be necessary, but this should be a last resort.

Technology plays a vital role in modern patient billing and collections. Electronic health records (EHR) systems streamline the entire process, from patient registration to final payment. EHRs can automate many tasks, such as insurance verification, coding, and claim submission, reducing the likelihood of errors and speeding up the billing cycle. Additionally, patient portals allow patients to access their billing information, make payments, and communicate with the billing department, enhancing transparency and convenience.

Training and education are ongoing needs in inpatient billing and collections. The healthcare landscape is constantly evolving, with changes in insurance policies, coding standards, and regulatory requirements. Regular training sessions for billing staff ensure that they stay current with these changes and maintain a high level of proficiency. Encouraging a culture of continuous improvement and providing resources for professional development can lead to more efficient and effective billing operations.

Patient satisfaction is closely tied to the billing experience. Transparent, accurate, and timely billing practices can enhance patient trust and loyalty. Conversely, billing errors, unexpected charges, and poor communication can lead to frustration and dissatisfaction. By prioritizing clear communication, accuracy, and empathy, healthcare providers can create a positive billing experience supporting patient satisfaction.

In summary, patient billing and collections are multifaceted processes that require meticulous attention to detail, effective communication, and a compassionate approach. From accurate patient registration to efficient coding and claims submission, each step plays a crucial role in ensuring financial stability for the healthcare provider and satisfaction for the patient. Leveraging technology, investing in training, and fostering a patient-centred approach can lead to successful billing and collections operations.

Case Studies and Scenarios

Case Study 1: The Overlooked Insurance Policy

A small clinic in a rural area faced a significant financial setback when they failed to verify a patient's insurance coverage before a major surgery.

The patient, believing they were covered, proceeded with the surgery. Post-operation, the clinic discovered that the insurance policy had lapsed, leaving the patient with a hefty bill and the clinic with a potential loss.

Case Study 2: The Coding Conundrum

A large urban hospital experienced a spike in claim denials due to incorrect coding. The billing department was overwhelmed, and the backlog of claims grew. After an internal audit, they discovered several coders were not up-to-date with the latest coding standards—the hospital invested in comprehensive training, which significantly reduced errors and improved reimbursement rates.

Case Study 3: The Compassionate Collection

A patient undergoing long-term treatment for a chronic illness accumulated a substantial balance. The billing department, recognizing the patient's financial hardship, offered a flexible payment plan. This approach helped patients manage their finances and ensured the hospital received timely payments.

Case Study 4: The Pre-Authorization Pitfall

A speciality clinic specializing in high-cost treatments faced frequent delays in reimbursement due to a lack of pre-authorization. By implementing a robust pre-authorization process, the clinic ensured that all necessary approvals were obtained before treatment, leading to faster reimbursements and improved cash flow.

Case Study 5: The Transparent Billing Triumph

A mid-sized healthcare provider revamped their billing statements to be more transparent and detailed. Patients received clear breakdowns of charges, insurance payments, and their responsibilities. This transparency led to fewer billing disputes and higher patient satisfaction.

Case Study 6: The EHR Revolution

A community health centre transitioned from paper to electronic health records (EHR) systems. This change streamlined their billing process, reduced errors, and improved efficiency. The centre saw a significant reduction in claim denials and faster reimbursement times.

Case Study 7: The Insurance Verification Victory

A pediatric clinic implemented a rigorous insurance verification process during patient registration. This proactive approach ensured that all services provided were covered, reducing the number of denied claims and improving the clinic's financial stability.

Case Study 8: The Patient Portal Success

A multi-specialty practice introduced a patient portal that allowed patients to view their billing information, make payments, and communicate with the billing department. This innovation increased patient engagement, timely payments, and reduced administrative workload.

Case Study 9: The Collections Agency Dilemma

A dental practice faced challenges with overdue accounts and decided to partner with a collections agency. While this approach recovered some outstanding balances, it also led to patient dissatisfaction. The practice learned the importance of balancing collections efforts with maintaining patient relationships.

Case Study 10: The Training Turnaround

A regional hospital invested in regular training sessions for their billing staff to update them on the latest insurance policies and coding standards. This investment paid off, as the hospital saw a marked improvement in claim accuracy and reduced denials.

Case Study 11: The Financial Counseling Initiative

A cancer treatment centre introduced financial counselling services for patients. Counselors helped patients understand their insurance coverage, potential out-of-pocket costs, and available financial assistance programs. This initiative improved patient satisfaction and reduced the number of unpaid bills.

Case Study 12: The Automated Billing System

A private practice adopted an automated billing system that integrated with their EHR. This system streamlined the billing process, from claim submission to payment posting, reducing manual errors and speeding up the revenue cycle.

Case Study 13: The Detailed Statement Strategy

A cardiology clinic sent detailed billing statements explaining each charge and insurance adjustment. This transparency helped patients understand their bills better and led to fewer disputes and faster payments.

Case Study 14: The Proactive Follow-Up

A physical therapy centre implemented a proactive follow-up system for overdue accounts. Gentle reminders and follow-up calls were made to patients with outstanding balances. This approach improved collections without damaging patient relationships.

Case Study 15: The Flexible Payment Plan

A mental health clinic offered flexible payment plans to patients facing financial difficulties. This compassionate approach ensured that patients continued to receive necessary care while managing their financial obligations.

Case Study 16: The Insurance Denial Appeal

A surgical centre faced a high rate of insurance denials for a specific procedure. They established a dedicated team to handle denial appeals, providing detailed documentation and justifications. This effort resulted in a higher success rate for appeals and improved revenue.

CHAPTER 6

EXAM PREPARATION TACTICS

Understanding the CPC Exam

The Certified Professional Coder (CPC) exam is a crucial milestone for those aspiring to excel in the medical coding field. This exam, administered by the American Academy of Professional Coders (AAPC), tests a candidate's knowledge and proficiency in medical coding, ensuring they are well-equipped to handle the complexities of the healthcare industry. The CPC exam is not just a test of memorization but a comprehensive assessment of one's ability to apply coding principles in real-world scenarios. Understanding the structure, content, and strategies for success is essential for anyone preparing to take this exam.

The CPC exam consists of multiple-choice questions that cover a wide range of topics, including medical terminology, anatomy, coding guidelines, and specific coding scenarios. It is designed to evaluate a candidate's ability to accurately code medical procedures and diagnoses using the Current Procedural Terminology (CPT), International Classification of Diseases (ICD), and Healthcare Common Procedure Coding System (HCPCS) codes. The exam is divided into sections, each focusing on different aspects of medical coding, such as evaluation and management, surgery, radiology, pathology, and medicine. This comprehensive approach ensures that candidates understand the coding process and can handle various coding challenges.

Preparation for the CPC exam requires a thorough understanding of the coding guidelines and the ability to apply them accurately. This involves studying the CPT, ICD, and HCPCS manuals and familiarizing oneself with the specific coding rules and conventions. Practice exams and coding exercises are invaluable tools for reinforcing this knowledge and building confidence. Additionally, attending coding courses or workshops can provide structured learning and expert guidance, helping candidates grasp complex concepts and stay updated with the latest coding changes.

Time management is a critical factor in successfully passing the CPC exam. With a limited amount of time to answer each question, candidates must be able to quickly and accurately identify the correct codes and apply them to the given scenarios. Developing effective test-taking strategies, such as reading the questions carefully, eliminating incorrect answers, and pacing oneself throughout the exam, can significantly improve one's chances of success. Staying calm and focused during the exam is also important, as stress and anxiety can hinder performance.

The CPC exam is not just a test of knowledge but a demonstration of one's ability to think critically and apply coding principles in real-world situations. This requires a deep understanding of medical terminology, anatomy, and coding guidelines and the ability to interpret and analyze medical records. Candidates must be able to accurately code complex medical procedures and diagnoses, ensuring that they meet the requirements of insurance companies and regulatory agencies. This level of expertise is essential for maintaining the integrity of the healthcare system and ensuring that patients receive the appropriate care and reimbursement.

In addition to technical knowledge, the CPC exam also assesses a candidate's ethical and professional standards. Medical coders play a crucial role in the healthcare industry, and their work directly impacts patient care and financial outcomes. Therefore, coders must adhere to the highest accuracy, integrity, and confidentiality standards. The CPC exam includes questions on coding ethics and compliance, ensuring that candidates understand the importance of ethical coding practices and are committed to upholding these standards.

Passing the CPC exam is a significant achievement that opens up numerous career opportunities in the medical coding field. Certified Professional Coders are in high demand, and healthcare providers, insurance companies, and regulatory agencies value their expertise. With a CPC certification, coders can pursue various roles, such as coding specialists, auditors, and educators. This certification also provides a solid foundation for further professional development and advancement in the healthcare industry.

Becoming a Certified Professional Coder requires dedication, hard work, and a commitment to continuous learning. The CPC exam is challenging, but with the proper preparation and mindset, candidates can succeed and embark on a rewarding career in medical coding. By understanding the structure and content of the exam, developing effective study strategies, and staying focused and motivated, aspiring coders can confidently tackle the CPC exam and achieve their professional goals.

One of the critical aspects of preparing for the CPC exam is mastering the use of coding manuals. The CPT, ICD, and HCPCS manuals are extensive, and knowing how to navigate them efficiently is crucial. Candidates should become familiar with the layout and organization of these manuals and the specific coding conventions and guidelines that apply to each section. Practising real-world coding scenarios can help candidates develop the skills to locate and use the correct codes during the exam quickly.

Another critical factor in exam preparation is understanding the common pitfalls and mistakes in medical coding. Errors such as upcoding, undercoding, and incorrect code selection can significantly affect patient care and reimbursement. Candidates can improve their accuracy and confidence by studying examples of common coding errors and learning how to avoid them. Understanding the rationale behind coding guidelines and conventions can help candidates make informed decisions when faced with complex or ambiguous coding scenarios.

The CPC exam also includes questions on medical billing and reimbursement, which are essential components of the coding process. Candidates should have a solid understanding of the various healthcare payment systems and reimbursement methodologies, as well as the rules and regulations governing billing practices. This knowledge is critical for ensuring that coded claims are accurate and compliant with payer requirements and maximizing reimbursement for healthcare providers.

In addition to technical skills, successful medical coders must possess strong analytical and problem-solving abilities. The CPC exam tests a candidate's ability to interpret and analyze medical records, identify relevant information, and apply the appropriate codes. This requires a keen attention to detail and the ability to think critically and logically. Developing these skills through practice and experience is essential for success on the exam and in the coding profession.

The role of a Certified Professional Coder extends beyond simply assigning codes to medical procedures and diagnoses. Coders play a vital role in the healthcare system, ensuring that medical records are accurate, complete, and compliant with regulatory requirements. They also contribute to the financial health of healthcare organizations by ensuring that coded claims are processed correctly and efficiently. As such, coders must be knowledgeable about healthcare laws and regulations and the ethical standards that govern their profession.

Ethical coding practices are a fundamental aspect of the CPC exam. Candidates must demonstrate an understanding of the principles of ethical coding, including accuracy, integrity, and confidentiality. This includes adhering to coding guidelines and conventions, avoiding fraudulent or deceptive coding practices, and maintaining the confidentiality of patient information. By upholding these ethical standards, coders help to ensure the integrity of the healthcare system and protect the rights and privacy of patients.

The CPC exam is a rigorous and challenging assessment, but it is also an opportunity for candidates to demonstrate their expertise and commitment to the medical coding profession. By thoroughly preparing for the exam, candidates can build the knowledge and skills needed to succeed and achieve their certification. This certification validates their coding proficiency and opens up many career opportunities in the healthcare industry.

Certified Professional Coders are highly valued for their expertise and play a critical role in the healthcare system. With a CPC certification, coders can pursue various career paths, including coding specialist, coding auditor, and coding educator. They can also work in multiple healthcare settings, such as hospitals, physician practices, insurance companies, and government agencies. The demand for skilled medical coders continues to grow, making this a rewarding and stable career choice.

Achieving CPC certification is a significant milestone that requires dedication, hard work, and a commitment to continuous learning. The journey to becoming a Certified Professional Coder is challenging, but with the proper preparation and mindset, candidates can succeed and make a meaningful impact in the healthcare industry. By mastering the coding guidelines, developing effective test-taking strategies, and upholding ethical standards, aspiring coders can confidently tackle the CPC exam and embark on a fulfilling and rewarding career in medical coding.

Creating an Effective Study Plan

A practical study plan is essential for anyone aiming to succeed academically or professionally. The process involves more than just setting aside time for studying; it requires a strategic approach considering individual learning styles, goals, and available resources. A well-structured study plan can help manage time efficiently, reduce stress, and improve learning outcomes. By understanding the critical components of an effective study plan, individuals can tailor their approach to meet their specific needs and maximize their potential.

The first step in creating an effective study plan is to set clear and achievable goals. These goals should be specific, measurable, attainable, relevant, and time-bound (SMART). For instance, instead of setting a vague goal like "study more," one might set a goal to "study for two hours every evening from 6 PM to 8 PM for the next month." This specificity level helps create a clear roadmap and provides a sense of direction. Additionally, breaking down larger goals into smaller, manageable tasks can make the process less overwhelming and more achievable.

Once goals are established, assessing one's current schedule and identifying available time slots for studying is essential. This involves closely examining daily routines, work commitments, and other responsibilities. Individuals can allocate specific periods for focused study sessions by identifying pockets of free time. It's also crucial to consider personal energy levels and peak productivity times. Some people may be more alert and focused in the morning, while others prefer studying in the evening. Aligning study sessions with these peak times can enhance concentration and retention.

Another critical aspect of an effective study plan is to create a conducive study environment. This means finding a quiet, comfortable, and well-lit space without distractions. Having all necessary materials and resources readily available can minimize interruptions and help maintain focus. Additionally, it's essential to establish a routine and stick to it as consistently as possible. Consistency helps to build good study habits and reinforces the importance of the study plan.

Incorporating various study techniques can also enhance the effectiveness of a study plan. Different subjects and types of material may require different approaches. For example, visual learners might benefit from using diagrams, charts, and flashcards, while auditory learners might prefer listening to lectures or discussing concepts with peers. Active learning techniques can also improve understanding and retention, such as summarizing information in one's own words, teaching the material to someone else, or applying concepts to real-world scenarios.

Various study techniques are essential for catering to different learning styles and enhancing retention. Visual learners might benefit from creating mind maps, diagrams, or flashcards to visualize information. Auditory learners could find it helpful to listen to recorded lectures, engage in discussions, or use mnemonic devices that involve sound.

 Kinesthetic learners, who learn best through hands-on activities, might prefer to engage in experiments, simulations, or role-playing exercises. By diversifying study methods, individuals can find the best techniques and keep their study sessions engaging.

Monitoring progress and adjusting as needed is another critical aspect of an effective study plan. Regularly reviewing goals and assessing whether they are being met can help identify areas needing improvement. If specific strategies or techniques are not working, it's essential to be flexible and willing to try new approaches. Seeking feedback from teachers, mentors, or peers can also provide valuable insights and help to refine the study plan.

Creating an effective study plan requires a thoughtful and strategic approach. By setting clear goals, assessing available time, creating a conducive study environment, incorporating various study techniques, taking regular breaks, and monitoring progress, individuals can develop a plan tailored to their specific needs and goals. This structured approach can help to manage time more efficiently, reduce stress, and improve overall learning outcomes.

A detailed explanation of the topic involves understanding the nuances and intricacies of each component of the study plan. Setting SMART goals is a foundational step that provides clarity and direction. Specific goals eliminate ambiguity and provide a clear target for which to aim. Measurable goals allow tracking progress and assessing whether the objectives are being met. Attainable goals ensure the targets are realistic and achievable within the given timeframe. Relevant goals align with broader academic or professional aspirations, ensuring that the effort invested is meaningful. Time-bound goals create a sense of urgency and help to prioritize tasks effectively.

Assessing one's current schedule involves thoroughly examining daily routines and commitments. This step requires honesty and self-awareness to identify potential time-wasters and areas where time can be better utilized. Individuals can see where study sessions can be integrated by visualizing the daily schedule, such as a timetable or calendar. It's also important to consider personal preferences and energy levels when scheduling study sessions. Aligning study times with periods of peak productivity can enhance focus and retention.

Creating a conducive study environment is crucial for maintaining concentration and minimizing distractions. This involves selecting a quiet and comfortable space free from interruptions. Ensuring that all necessary materials, such as textbooks, notebooks, and stationery, are readily available can help to minimize disruptions. Personalizing the study space with motivational quotes or organizing it to promote efficiency can also contribute to a more productive study session. For instance, keeping the study area tidy and well-organized can reduce the time spent searching for materials and help maintain focus.

Active learning techniques are particularly effective for deepening understanding and improving retention. Summarizing information in one's own words forces the brain to process and internalize the material. Teaching the material to someone else, whether it's a peer, a family member, or even an imaginary audience, can reinforce understanding and highlight gaps in knowledge. Applying concepts to real-world scenarios or solving practical problems can also help to solidify understanding and make the material more relevant and memorable.

Regular breaks are a crucial component of any effective study plan. The brain's ability to maintain high focus and concentration levels diminishes, making taking short breaks to recharge essential. Techniques like the Pomodoro Technique, which involves studying for 25 minutes followed by a 5-minute break, can help to maintain focus and prevent burnout. During these breaks, engaging in activities that promote relaxation and mental rejuvenation, such as stretching, walking, or practising mindfulness, can be beneficial. Longer breaks should also be scheduled to allow for leisure activities and social interactions, which are essential for overall well-being and mental health.

Monitoring progress and adjusting as needed is another critical aspect of an effective study plan. Regularly reviewing goals and assessing whether they are being met can help identify areas needing improvement. If specific strategies or techniques are not working, it's essential to be flexible and willing to try new approaches. Seeking feedback from teachers, mentors, or peers can also provide valuable insights and help to refine the study plan. Keeping a study journal can help track progress, reflect on what works and doesn't, and make necessary adjustments.

In addition to these core components, it's essential to consider the role of motivation and mindset in the effectiveness of a study plan. Maintaining a positive and growth-oriented mindset can help to overcome challenges and setbacks. Setting up a system of rewards and incentives for achieving study goals can also boost motivation and make the process more enjoyable. Celebrating small victories and acknowledging progress can help to maintain momentum and build confidence.

A practical study plan is not a one-size-fits-all solution but a personalized approach considering individual needs, preferences, and goals. By setting clear and achievable goals, assessing available time, creating a conducive study environment, incorporating various study techniques, taking regular breaks, monitoring progress, and maintaining a positive mindset, individuals can develop a study plan that maximizes their potential and leads to academic and professional success.

Test-Taking Strategies

Test-taking can be a daunting experience for many, often filled with anxiety and uncertainty. However, it can become a manageable and rewarding process with the right strategies. The key lies in preparation, understanding the test format, and employing effective techniques during the exam. These strategies help maximize performance, reduce stress, and boost confidence. Students can navigate tests more efficiently and achieve better results by approaching tests with a well-thought-out plan.

Preparation is the cornerstone of effective test-taking. It begins long before the test day and involves consistent study habits, a thorough understanding of the material, and regular review sessions. Creating a study schedule that allocates specific times for different subjects or topics can help cover all necessary content without feeling overwhelmed. Starting this process early is essential, allowing ample time to absorb and understand the material rather than cramming it at the last minute. Various study techniques can enhance retention and understanding, such as summarizing notes, creating flashcards, and practising past papers.

Understanding the test format is another crucial aspect of preparation. Different tests have different structures, and knowing what to expect can significantly impact performance. For instance, multiple-choice tests require a different approach compared to essay-based exams. Familiarizing oneself with the format, types of questions, and time constraints can help devise effective strategies. Practice tests can be instrumental in this regard, as they provide a realistic exam simulation and help identify areas that need improvement.

During the test, time management is critical. It's essential to allocate time wisely, ensuring that each question or section receives adequate attention. Starting with more straightforward questions can help build confidence and secure quick points, while more challenging questions can be tackled later. It's also essential to monitor the clock and pace oneself accordingly. If a question seems too complicated, it's better to move on and return to it later rather than getting stuck and wasting valuable time.

Reading instructions carefully is another essential strategy. Misinterpreting a question or missing specific instructions can lead to unnecessary mistakes. Taking a few moments to read and understand the instructions can save time and prevent errors. For multiple-choice questions, eliminating incorrect options can increase the chances of selecting the correct answer. In essay-based exams, outlining the main points before writing can help organize thoughts and present a coherent argument.

Maintaining a calm and focused mindset during the test is crucial. Anxiety can cloud judgment and hinder performance, so staying composed is essential. Deep breathing exercises, positive self-talk, and visualization techniques can help manage stress. Short breaks can also provide a mental reset and improve concentration if allowed. Staying hydrated and having a healthy snack before the test is essential to ensure optimal physical and psychological functioning.

After the test, reviewing the answers, if time permits, can help catch any mistakes or overlooked questions. It's essential to approach this review critically, ensuring that all questions have been answered and the answers are accurate. For essay-based exams, checking for grammatical errors, clarity, and coherence can enhance the overall quality of the response.

In addition to these general strategies, specific techniques can be employed for different types of tests. For multiple-choice tests, the process of elimination can be particularly effective. Systematically ruling out incorrect options increases the chances of selecting the correct answer. It's also helpful to look for keywords or phrases in the question that can provide clues to the correct answer. For true/false questions, paying attention to absolute terms like "always" or "never" can be helpful, as these statements are often false.

For essay-based exams, planning and organization are key. Starting with a clear thesis statement and outlining the main points can provide a roadmap for the essay. Each paragraph should focus on a single point supported by evidence and examples. Transition words and phrases can help in maintaining a logical flow and coherence. It's essential to stay on topic and avoid unnecessary tangents. Concluding the essay with a strong summary of the main points can leave a positive impression on the examiner.

For problem-solving tests, such as those in mathematics or science, showing all steps and workings is essential. Even if the final answer is incorrect, partial credit can often be awarded for the correct method. It's also helpful to double-check calculations and ensure that all units and measurements are accurate. For open-ended questions, a clear and concise explanation of the reasoning process can demonstrate a thorough understanding of the material.

In language tests, such as those assessing reading comprehension or writing skills, attention to grammar, punctuation, and spelling is crucial. Reading the passage or prompt carefully and identifying the main ideas can help answer questions accurately. Planning and organizing the response for writing tasks can enhance clarity and coherence. It's essential to stay within the word limit and avoid unnecessary repetition.

In conclusion, effective test-taking strategies involve:

- A combination of preparation.
- Understanding the test format.
- Time management.
- A careful reading of instructions.
- Maintaining a calm mindset.
- Employing specific techniques for different types of tests.

By adopting these strategies, students can confidently approach tests and achieve their best performance. It's essential to remember that test-taking is a skill that can be developed and refined over time. Each test provides an opportunity to learn and improve, and by reflecting on past experiences, students can identify what works best for them and make necessary adjustments.

One often overlooked aspect of test preparation is the importance of a healthy lifestyle. Adequate sleep, regular exercise, and a balanced diet significantly affect cognitive function and overall well-being. Sleep, in particular, is crucial for memory consolidation and mental clarity.

Ensuring a good night's sleep before the test can substantially affect performance. Regular physical activity helps reduce stress and improve concentration, while a nutritious diet provides the necessary energy and nutrients for optimal brain function.

Another valuable strategy is to form study groups with peers. Collaborative learning can provide different perspectives and insights, making the study process more engaging and effective. Group discussions can help clarify doubts, reinforce concepts, and share valuable resources. However, ensuring the group remains focused and productive is essential, as well as avoiding distractions and staying on track with the study goals.

Mindfulness and relaxation techniques can also be beneficial in managing test anxiety. Practices such as meditation, deep breathing exercises, and progressive muscle relaxation can help calm the mind and reduce stress. These techniques can be incorporated into the daily routine and used during the test to maintain composure and focus.

It's also helpful to seek support from teachers, mentors, or counsellors. They can provide valuable guidance, resources, and encouragement. Teachers can offer insights into the test format, essential topics, and effective study strategies. Mentors and counsellors can provide emotional support and help develop a positive mindset.

For students with specific learning needs or disabilities, exploring available accommodations and support services is essential. Many educational institutions offer accommodations such as extended time, separate testing environments, or assistive technology. Understanding and utilizing these resources can help level the playing field and ensure all students have an equal opportunity to succeed.

In the digital age, numerous online resources and tools are available to aid in test preparation. Educational websites, online courses, and mobile apps offer interactive, engaging study and practice methods. These resources can provide additional practice questions, tutorials, and feedback, helping students to reinforce their understanding and track their progress.

Maintaining a positive attitude and staying motivated throughout preparation is also essential. Setting realistic goals and celebrating small achievements can help maintain momentum and build confidence. Visualizing success and focusing on the effort rather than the outcome can create a more positive and empowering mindset.

Lastly, it's essential to remember that tests are just one aspect of the educational journey. While important, they do not define a student's worth or potential. It's essential to keep things in perspective and not let the pressure of tests overshadow the broader goals of learning and personal growth. Embracing a growth mindset, where challenges are seen as opportunities for learning and improvement, can lead to a more fulfilling and successful academic experience.

Students can approach tests more confidently and effectively by integrating these strategies into their routines. The test-taking journey becomes about achieving high scores, developing valuable skills, building resilience, and fostering a lifelong love for learning.

Exam Success Mindset

Success in exams often hinges on more than just understanding the material; it requires cultivating the right mindset. This mindset encompasses a blend of confidence, resilience, and strategic thinking. Developing such a mindset can transform how students approach their studies and, ultimately, their performance on exam day.

The journey begins with self-belief. Confidence is not about knowing everything but trusting in one's ability to learn and apply knowledge effectively. This trust is built through consistent effort and recognizing small victories along the way. For instance, mastering a challenging concept or solving a complex problem can boost confidence significantly. Celebrating these milestones is essential, no matter how minor they may seem.

Resilience is another critical component. Exams can be stressful, and setbacks are inevitable. Whether a poor score on a practice test or difficulty understanding a particular topic, resilience helps students bounce back and continue their preparation with renewed vigour. This resilience is fostered by maintaining a positive attitude and viewing challenges as opportunities for growth rather than insurmountable obstacles.

Strategic thinking involves planning and prioritizing study efforts. It's about identifying the most critical areas to focus on and allocating time efficiently. This requires a thorough understanding of the exam format and the weightage of different sections. Creating a study schedule that balances various subjects and includes regular breaks can prevent burnout and ensure a more productive study session.

A detailed explanation of the exam success mindset involves delving deeper into these components. Confidence can be nurtured through various techniques. Visualization is one such method. By picturing oneself successfully answering questions and performing well, students can create a mental blueprint for success. This technique can reduce anxiety and build a positive outlook towards exams.

Another technique is positive self-talk. Replacing negative thoughts with affirmations like "I am prepared" or "I can handle this" can shift the mindset from doubt to determination. It's also helpful to surround oneself with supportive peers and mentors who can provide encouragement and constructive feedback.

Resilience can be developed through mindfulness practices. Meditation and deep breathing can help manage stress and maintain focus. These practices train the mind to stay calm under pressure, which is invaluable during exams. Setting realistic goals and breaking down study material into manageable chunks can make the preparation process less overwhelming.

Strategic thinking involves not just planning but also adaptability. It's essential to regularly assess one's progress and adjust the study plan as needed. For example, if a topic proves more challenging than anticipated, it may require additional time and resources. Conversely, if a topic is mastered quickly, the saved time can be reallocated to other areas.

A comprehensive review of the exam success mindset reveals its multifaceted nature. Confidence, resilience, and strategic thinking are interlinked and reinforce each other. Confidence grows with resilience, as overcoming challenges builds self-belief. Strategic thinking supports resilience by providing a clear plan and reducing uncertainty, which can be a significant source of stress.

Consider the story of a student named Alex. Alex struggled with math and often felt overwhelmed by the subject. However, by adopting a success mindset, Alex transformed his approach. He started by setting small, achievable goals, such as mastering one concept at a time. Each success, no matter how small, boosted his confidence.

Alex also practised visualization, picturing himself solving math problems with ease. This mental rehearsal reduced his anxiety and made him more comfortable with the subject. When faced with setbacks, such as a low score on a practice test, Alex used positive self-talk to stay motivated. He reminded himself that setbacks were part of the learning process and not a reflection of his abilities.

To build resilience, Alex incorporated mindfulness practices into his routine. He spent a few minutes each day meditating and practising deep breathing exercises. These practices helped him stay calm and focused despite high pressure. Alex also created a study schedule that balanced his time between different subjects and included regular breaks to prevent burnout.

Strategic thinking played a crucial role in Alex's success. He analyzed the exam format and identified the areas that required the most attention. By prioritizing these areas, he made his study sessions more efficient. Alex also regularly assessed his progress and adjusted his study plan as needed. This adaptability ensured that he was always on track and made the most of his study time.

Alex's story illustrates how the exam success mindset can transform a student's approach to studying and significantly improve their performance. Students can tackle exams with a positive attitude and a clear plan by building confidence, resilience, and strategic thinking.

The exam success mindset is not just about passing exams; it's about developing valuable skills and attitudes in all areas of life. Confidence, resilience, and strategic thinking are essential for personal and professional growth. Students can achieve their academic goals and prepare for future challenges by cultivating these qualities.

CHAPTER 7

LANDING YOUR FIRST CODING JOB

Crafting a Winning Resume

Crafting a resume that stands out in a sea of applicants is both an art and a science. It's not just about listing your qualifications and experiences; it's about presenting them in a way that captures the attention of hiring managers and showcases your unique value. A well-crafted resume can be the key to unlocking new career opportunities, making it essential to understand the nuances of creating one that truly shines.

The first step in crafting a winning resume is understanding its purpose. A resume is a marketing tool designed to sell your skills, experiences, and potential to a prospective employer. It's your first impression; as the saying goes, you never get a second chance to make a first impression. Therefore, ensuring that your resume is accurate, comprehensive, engaging, and easy to read is crucial.

Begin by selecting the right format. There are several resume formats, including chronological, functional, and combination. The most common chronological format lists your work experience in reverse chronological order. This format is ideal for individuals with a strong work history in a specific field. The functional format, on the other hand, focuses on skills and experiences rather than chronological work history. This format suits those with gaps in their employment history or those looking to change careers. The combination format merges elements of both chronological and functional formats, providing a balanced approach that highlights skills and work experience.

Once you've chosen the appropriate format, it's time to focus on the content. Start with a compelling summary or objective statement. This section should be a brief, powerful introduction that highlights your essential qualifications and career goals. It should grab the reader's attention and make them want to learn more about you. Avoid generic statements and tailor this section to the specific job you're applying for.

Next, detail your work experience. Use bullet points to list your responsibilities and achievements for each position. Be specific and quantify your accomplishments whenever possible. For example, instead of saying, "Managed a team," say, "Managed a team of 10 employees, increasing productivity by 20%." This provides concrete evidence of your abilities and makes your resume more engaging and impactful.

Education is another critical component of your resume. List your educational background chronologically, starting with your most recent degree. Include the institution's name, the degree obtained, and attendance dates. If you have relevant coursework or honours, include those as well.

Skills are an essential part of any resume. Create a separate section to list your relevant skills, both hard and soft. Hard skills are specific, teachable abilities such as proficiency in a foreign language or expertise in a particular software. Soft skills, on the other hand, are interpersonal attributes like communication, teamwork, and problem-solving. Tailor this section to the job you're applying for, emphasizing the most relevant skills.

In addition to the main sections, consider including additional sections that can set you apart from other candidates. These might include certifications, professional affiliations, volunteer work, or publications. Each section provides an opportunity to showcase your unique qualifications and experiences.

The design and layout of your resume are just as important as the content. Use a clean, professional layout with plenty of white space. Choose a simple, easy-to-read font and use consistent formatting throughout. Avoid using excessive colours or graphics, which can be distracting and make your resume look unprofessional.

Proofreading is a critical final step in the resume-crafting process. Even a small typo or grammatical error can negatively impact a potential employer. Take the time to review your resume for any mistakes carefully, and consider asking a friend or mentor to review it.

A winning resume is more than just a list of qualifications and experiences. It's a strategic document designed to showcase your unique value and make a compelling case for why you're the best candidate for the job. By understanding the purpose of a resume, choosing the right format, and focusing on content, design, and proofreading, you can create a resume that stands out and opens doors to new career opportunities.

When it comes to the detailed explanation of crafting a winning resume, it's essential to delve deeper into each component. For instance, the summary or objective statement should be more than just a brief introduction. It should encapsulate your professional identity and career aspirations in a way that resonates with the hiring manager. Think of it as your elevator pitch – a concise, compelling narrative that highlights your most significant achievements and sets the tone for the rest of your resume.

In the work experience section, using action verbs can make a significant difference. Words like "developed," "implemented," "managed," and "led" convey a sense of initiative and accomplishment. Pair these action verbs with quantifiable results to create a powerful impact. For example, "Implemented a new inventory management system, reducing stock discrepancies by 30%" is far more compelling than a vague description of duties.

The education section should not be overlooked, especially for recent graduates or those with relevant academic achievements. Including details such as your GPA (if it's impressive), relevant coursework, research projects, and academic honours can provide additional context and demonstrate your commitment to your field. Focusing on professional development courses, certifications, and continuing education can be equally valuable for those further in their careers.

When listing your skills, balancing hard and soft skills is essential. Hard skills, such as proficiency in specific software, technical abilities, or language fluency, are often easier to quantify and demonstrate. Soft skills, like leadership, communication, and adaptability, are equally important but can be more challenging to convey. Use specific examples from your work experience to illustrate these skills in action. For instance, instead of simply stating "strong communication skills," you might say, "Led weekly team meetings to ensure clear communication and alignment on project goals."

Additional sections, such as certifications, professional affiliations, volunteer work, or publications, can provide a more comprehensive picture of your qualifications and interests. Certifications demonstrate your commitment to professional development and can set you apart in fields where specific credentials are highly valued. Professional affiliations show your engagement with your industry and can indicate a network of contacts and resources. Volunteer work can highlight your dedication to community service and provide examples of transferable skills—publications, whether articles, research papers, or books, can establish your expertise and thought leadership.

The design and layout of your resume should reflect your professionalism and attention to detail. Use a clean, modern design with consistent formatting. Avoid overly complex layouts or excessive use of colours and graphics, which can distract from the content. Instead, focus on creating a visually appealing document that is easy to read and navigate. Use headings and subheadings to organize the information, and ensure plenty of white space to prevent the resume from cluttering.

Proofreading is an essential step that cannot be overstated. Even minor errors can detract from the overall impression of your resume. Carefully review your document for spelling, grammar, and punctuation errors. Use tools like spell and grammar checks, but don't rely on them entirely. Reading your resume out loud can help you catch mistakes you might miss when reading silently.

Additionally, having a trusted friend, mentor, or professional review your resume can provide valuable feedback and catch errors you might have overlooked.

Incorporating keywords from the job description into your resume can also improve your chances of getting noticed. Many companies use applicant tracking systems (ATS) to screen resumes before they reach a human recruiter. By including relevant keywords and phrases from the job posting, you can increase the likelihood that your resume will pass through these automated filters. However, use these keywords naturally and in context rather than simply stuffing them into your resume.

Tailoring your resume for each job application is another crucial strategy. While it may be tempting to use a one-size-fits-all approach, customizing your resume for each position can significantly improve your chances of success. Highlight the experiences and skills most relevant to the job, and adjust your summary or objective statement to align with the company's values and goals. This demonstrates your genuine interest in the position and shows that you have taken the time to understand what the employer is looking for.

Networking can also play a vital role in the job search process. While a well-crafted resume is essential, building relationships with professionals in your industry can open doors and provide valuable opportunities. Attend industry events, join professional organizations, and connect with colleagues and mentors. These connections can provide insights into job openings, offer recommendations, and even help you get your resume in front of the right people.

In the digital age, having an online presence is increasingly important. Consider creating a professional LinkedIn profile that complements your resume. Ensure your profile is complete, up-to-date, and reflects your professional brand. Use a professional photo, write a compelling headline and summary, and include detailed information about your work experience, education, and skills. Engage with your network by sharing relevant content, participating in discussions, and connecting with industry professionals.

A winning resume is a dynamic document that evolves with your career. Regularly update your resume to reflect new experiences, skills, and accomplishments. This ensures that you are always prepared for new opportunities and allows you to reflect on your professional growth and achievements.

Crafting a stand-out resume requires strategic thinking, attention to detail, and a deep understanding of what employers seek. By focusing on the critical components of a resume, tailoring it to each job application, and leveraging your network and online presence, you can create a powerful tool that opens doors to new career opportunities.

Networking and Finding Job Leads

Networking and finding job leads can feel like navigating a labyrinth, especially for beginners. The process is multifaceted, involving both strategic planning and spontaneous opportunities. Networking isn't just about collecting business cards or adding connections on LinkedIn; it's about building genuine relationships that can lead to career opportunities. Job leads, on the other hand, are the tangible outcomes of effective networking. They are the openings, referrals, and insider information that can give you a competitive edge in the job market.

Imagine walking into a room full of strangers at a professional event. The air is thick with anticipation, and you can almost hear the hum of potential connections waiting to be made. This is the essence of networking. It's about stepping out of your comfort zone and engaging with people who can influence your career trajectory. Every interaction promises a new opportunity, whether a casual conversation at a coffee shop or a formal introduction at a conference.

Networking is not a one-time event but a continuous process. It requires patience, persistence, and a genuine interest in others.

The key is to approach networking with an open mind and a willingness to give as much as you hope to receive. This means offering your expertise, sharing valuable information, and being a reliable contact for others. Doing so builds a network of trusted relationships that can support you throughout your career.

Finding job leads is the next step in the process. Once you've established a network, it's time to leverage those connections to uncover job opportunities. This involves more than asking for job openings; it's about being proactive and strategic. For instance, you might contact a contact in your network to inquire about potential openings at their company or ask for an introduction to someone in your desired field. The goal is to position yourself as a top candidate by tapping into the hidden job market—those positions that are not advertised publicly but are filled through referrals and recommendations.

Networking and finding job leads require effective communication, active listening, and strategic thinking. It's about knowing when to speak when to listen when to ask for help, and when to offer it. By mastering these skills, you can confidently navigate the job market and uncover opportunities that might remain hidden.

The art of networking lies in its subtlety. It's not about aggressively promoting yourself but about building meaningful connections. Start by identifying your goals. Are you looking to switch careers, climb the corporate ladder, or simply expand your professional circle? Knowing your objectives will help you target suitable events and people.

Attend industry conferences, seminars, and workshops. These gatherings are gold mines for networking. Engage in conversations, ask insightful questions, and exchange contact information. Follow up with a personalized message to reinforce the connection. Social media platforms like LinkedIn are also invaluable tools. Join relevant groups, participate in discussions, and share content that showcases your expertise.

Informational interviews are another powerful networking tool. Reach out to professionals in your field and request a brief meeting to learn about their career paths and insights. This not only expands your network but also provides valuable industry knowledge.

Finding job leads often involves a proactive approach. Regularly check job boards, company websites, and professional associations for openings. Set up job alerts to stay informed about new postings. However, the most effective job leads often come from within your network. Let your contacts know you're on the job hunt. They might have insider information about upcoming vacancies or can refer you to hiring managers.

Tailor your resume and cover letter for each application. Highlight your relevant skills and experiences, and demonstrate how you can add value to the organization. Prepare for interviews by researching the company and practising common interview questions. Show enthusiasm and confidence, and be ready to discuss how your background aligns with the job requirements.

Networking and finding job leads are intertwined processes. Effective networking can lead to valuable job leads, and pursuing job leads can expand your network. It's a dynamic cycle that requires continuous effort and adaptability. You can unlock a world of career opportunities by honing your networking skills and staying proactive in your job search.

Consider the story of Jane, a marketing professional looking to transition into a new industry. She started attending industry events and connecting with professionals on LinkedIn. These interactions taught her about a job opening at a company she admired. Jane contacted a contact she had met at a conference who worked at that company and asked for an informational interview. She expressed interest in the position during the meeting and shared her resume. Her contact was impressed, and she was referred to the hiring manager. Jane's proactive networking efforts paid off, and she landed the job.

Networking and finding job leads are about securing a job and building a sustainable career. By cultivating relationships and staying informed about industry trends, you position yourself as a valuable asset in the job market. The journey requires dedication, but the rewards are well worth the effort.

Interviewing Skills and Mock Interviews

Interviewing skills are essential for anyone looking to secure a job, advance their career, or network effectively. The ability to present oneself confidently, answer questions thoughtfully, and engage with interviewers can make a significant difference in the outcome of an interview. This chapter delves into the nuances of interviewing skills and the importance of mock interviews in honing these abilities.

The first step in mastering interviewing skills is understanding the different types of interviews one might encounter. Traditional one-on-one interviews are common, but there are also panel, group, and virtual interviews. Each type requires a slightly different approach. For instance, a panel interview might involve multiple interviewers asking questions rapidly, requiring the candidate to maintain composure and address each person individually. On the other hand, a virtual interview demands proficiency with technology and the ability to convey enthusiasm and professionalism through a screen.

Preparation is crucial to success in any interview. Researching the company, understanding its culture, and familiarizing oneself with the job description are fundamental steps. This knowledge not only helps in answering questions more effectively but also demonstrates genuine interest in the position. Additionally, preparing answers to common interview questions can boost confidence. Questions like "Tell me about yourself," "What are your strengths and weaknesses?" and "Why do you want to work here?" are almost guaranteed to come up. Writing thoughtful, concise responses to these questions can set a candidate apart.

Body language plays a crucial role in interviews. Non-verbal cues such as eye contact, posture, and hand gestures can convey confidence and enthusiasm. Maintaining eye contact shows attentiveness and interest, while a firm handshake can leave a lasting positive impression. It's also important to be mindful of nervous habits, such as fidgeting or avoiding eye contact, as these can detract from the overall appearance.

Mock interviews are an invaluable tool for improving interviewing skills. They provide a safe environment to practice responses, receive feedback, and make adjustments. Conducting mock interviews with friends, family, or career coaches can help identify areas for improvement. Recording and reviewing these sessions can also be beneficial, allowing candidates to see themselves from an interviewer's perspective and make necessary changes.

Simulating actual interview conditions as closely as possible during a mock interview is essential. This includes dressing appropriately, using professional language, and treating the mock interview with the same seriousness as a real one. Feedback from mock interviews should be taken constructively. It's an opportunity to refine answers, improve body language, and build confidence.

One of the most challenging aspects of an interview is handling unexpected questions. These questions test a candidate's ability to think on their feet and handle pressure. Practising responses to various questions, including behavioural and situational ones, can help prepare for these moments. Behavioural questions often start with phrases like "Tell me about a time when..." and require candidates to provide specific examples from their past experiences. Situational questions, on the other hand, present hypothetical scenarios and ask how the candidate would handle them.

Effective communication is another critical component of successful interviewing. This includes not only verbal communication but also active listening. Answering questions clearly and concisely is essential, but so is listening carefully to the interviewer's questions and responding appropriately. It's also beneficial to ask thoughtful questions at the end of the interview. This demonstrates interest in the role and the company and can provide valuable insights into the job and the team.

Confidence is vital in any interview. Confidence comes from preparation, practice, and self-awareness. Knowing one's strengths and articulating them effectively can make a significant difference. It's also important to acknowledge areas for improvement and demonstrate a willingness to learn and grow. This balance of confidence and humility can leave a positive impression on interviewers.

In addition to traditional preparation methods, several techniques can help boost confidence and reduce anxiety before an interview. Visualization is one such technique. Candidates can build a positive mindset by imagining a successful interview and visualizing themselves answering questions confidently. Deep breathing exercises and mindfulness practices can help calm nerves and improve focus.

The STAR method is a valuable framework for answering behavioural questions. STAR stands for Situation, Task, Action, and Result. Candidates can provide clear, concise, and compelling responses by structuring answers. For example, if asked about a time when they faced a challenging situation, a candidate might describe the problem, explain the task they needed to accomplish, outline the actions they took, and highlight the positive results of their efforts.

Networking can also play a role in interview success. Building relationships with professionals in the industry can provide valuable insights and advice. Networking events, informational interviews, and professional associations are all opportunities to connect with others and learn from their experiences. These connections can also lead to job referrals and recommendations, which can be advantageous in the interview process.

Finally, it's essential to follow up after an interview. Sending the interviewer a thank-you email or note expresses gratitude for the opportunity and reinforces interest in the position. This small gesture can leave a lasting positive impression and set a candidate apart. Interview skills are not just about answering questions; they encompass a range of abilities that contribute to making a solid impression. One such ability is storytelling. Crafting compelling narratives about past experiences can make responses more engaging and memorable. Instead of simply stating that one has strong leadership skills, sharing a specific story that illustrates those skills in action can be far more impactful. This approach highlights competencies and provides a glimpse into the candidate's personality and values.

Another critical aspect is adaptability. Interviews can be unpredictable, and the ability to adapt to different situations and questions is invaluable. This might involve shifting gears when an interviewer changes the topic abruptly or handling technical difficulties during a virtual interview.

Demonstrating flexibility and a calm demeanour in the face of unexpected challenges can impress interviewers and show that the candidate can handle the pressures of the job.

Emotional intelligence also plays a significant role in interviews. Reading the room, understanding the interviewer's tone and body language, and responding appropriately can create a more positive interaction. This includes showing empathy, being respectful, and building rapport. For example, if an interviewer seems particularly interested in a specific aspect of the candidate's experience, elaborating on that topic can create a more engaging conversation.

It's also important to be authentic. While preparation and practice are crucial, authenticity should not be sacrificed. Interviewers can often tell when a candidate is being disingenuous or overly rehearsed. Being genuine and honest about one's experiences, strengths, and areas for growth can create a more authentic connection and leave a lasting impression.

In addition to verbal communication, written communication skills can be assessed during the interview. This might include writing samples, email correspondence, or even the thank-you note sent after the interview. Clear, concise, and professional written communication can reinforce a candidate's qualifications and attention to detail.

Cultural fit is another consideration for interviewers. Beyond assessing skills and experience, interviewers often look for candidates who align with the company's values and culture. This might involve questions about how the candidate handles teamwork, conflict, or work-life balance. Understanding the company's culture and providing examples of how one's values align with it can strengthen a candidate's position.

Mock interviews can also help candidates practice handling difficult questions or addressing potential red flags in their resume. For example, if there is a gap in employment or a career change, preparing a thoughtful explanation can help mitigate concerns. Being proactive in addressing these issues shows self-awareness and a willingness to be transparent.

The role of feedback in improving interviewing skills cannot be overstated. Constructive feedback from mock interviews, career coaches, or mentors can provide valuable insights and help identify areas for improvement.

It's essential to approach input with an open mind and a willingness to make adjustments. This iterative practice, feedback, and improvement process can lead to significant progress over time.

Incorporating humour, when appropriate, can also enhance the interview experience. A well-timed, light-hearted comment can break the ice and create a more relaxed atmosphere. However, gauging the interviewer's demeanour and ensuring that humour is used appropriately and professionally is essential.

Lastly, reflecting on past interview experiences can provide valuable lessons. Analyzing what went well and what could have been improved can inform future preparation and performance. Keeping a journal of interview experiences, including questions asked and responses given, can serve as a valuable reference for future interviews.

Mastering interviewing skills is a multifaceted endeavour involving preparation, practice, adaptability, and self-awareness. Mock interviews are a powerful tool, providing a safe space to refine skills and build confidence. Candidates can significantly enhance their chances of success by approaching interviews with preparation, authenticity, and emotional intelligence.

Negotiating Job Offers

Negotiating job offers can be daunting, especially for those new to the workforce or transitioning to a new career. The process involves more than just discussing salary; it encompasses a range of factors that can significantly impact one's professional and personal life. Understanding the nuances of negotiation can empower individuals to secure better terms and conditions, ultimately leading to greater job satisfaction and career growth.

The first step in negotiating a job offer is thorough preparation. Researching the industry standards for the role, understanding the company's compensation structure, and knowing one's worth in the job market is crucial. This information provides a solid foundation for making informed decisions and setting realistic expectations. Additionally, reflecting on personal priorities and career goals can help identify the most critical aspects of the offer. Salary may be the primary concern for some, while others might prioritize work-life balance, professional development opportunities, or benefits such as health insurance and retirement plans.

Effective communication is vital during the negotiation process. It's essential to approach the conversation confidently and professionally, clearly articulating one's value and the reasons for requesting specific terms. Using data and examples to support one's case can make the argument more compelling. For instance, highlighting relevant skills, experiences, and accomplishments that align with the job requirements can demonstrate why the candidate deserves a higher salary or additional benefits. It's also essential to listen actively and be open to the employer's perspective, as this can lead to a more collaborative and positive negotiation experience.

Timing plays a significant role in negotiations. Initiating the conversation at the right moment can increase the chances of a favourable outcome. Typically, the best time to negotiate is after receiving a formal job offer but before accepting it. This is when the employer has expressed interest in the candidate and is more likely to be flexible. However, it's essential to be mindful of the company's timeline and avoid delaying the process unnecessarily. Respecting the employer's time and showing enthusiasm for the role can help maintain a positive rapport throughout the negotiation.

Flexibility and creativity can also enhance the negotiation process. While salary is often the primary focus, many other aspects of a job offer can be negotiated. For example, candidates can discuss options such as signing bonuses, relocation assistance, flexible work schedules, remote work opportunities, additional vacation days, or professional development funding. Being open to alternative solutions and finding mutually beneficial arrangements can produce a more satisfactory outcome for both parties.

Understanding the employer's constraints and priorities can provide valuable insights during negotiations. Companies may have budget limitations or specific policies restricting their ability to meet certain requests. By acknowledging these constraints and proposing reasonable alternatives, candidates can demonstrate their willingness to work collaboratively and find solutions that align with the company's needs. This approach can also help build trust and strengthen the relationship with the employer.

It's crucial to approach negotiations with a positive and respectful attitude. While advocating for oneself is essential, it's equally important to maintain professionalism and avoid being aggressive or demanding. Expressing gratitude for the offer and showing appreciation for the opportunity can create a more amicable atmosphere. Additionally, being prepared to compromise and find common ground can lead to a more successful negotiation.

Once an agreement has been reached, it's crucial to get the final offer in writing. This ensures that both parties clearly understand the terms and conditions and can prevent any misunderstandings or discrepancies in the future.

Reviewing the written offer carefully and seeking clarification on any ambiguous points can provide peace of mind and ensure that all agreement aspects are accurately documented.

Negotiating job offers is a skill that can be developed and refined over time. By approaching the process with preparation, confidence, and a collaborative mindset, individuals can secure better terms and conditions that align with their career goals and personal priorities. This enhances job satisfaction and sets the stage for long-term professional growth and success.

In the detailed explanation of negotiating job offers, it's essential to delve deeper into specific strategies and techniques that can be employed to achieve favourable outcomes. One practical approach is to use the "anchoring" method, where the candidate sets the initial terms of the negotiation. By proposing a specific salary or benefits package, the candidate can influence the direction of the conversation and establish a reference point for further discussions. This approach can be beneficial when the employer has not provided a clear starting point for the negotiation.

Another technique is to leverage multiple offers or competing opportunities. If a candidate has received offers from other companies, they can use this information to strengthen their negotiating position. By highlighting other employers' interests, the candidate can create a sense of urgency and demonstrate their value in the job market. However, it's essential to approach this tactic cautiously, avoid appearing cautiously, and avoid appearing overly aggressive or manipulative.

Building rapport with the employer can also enhance the negotiation process. Establishing a positive relationship and demonstrating genuine interest in the company and the role can create a more collaborative atmosphere. This can be achieved by asking thoughtful questions, showing enthusiasm for the job, and being willing to contribute to the company's success. Building rapport can also help the candidate gain insights into the employer's priorities and constraints, which can inform their negotiation strategy.

Career Growth and Advancement

Navigating the career growth and advancement labyrinth can often feel like an intricate dance, where each step must be carefully calculated and executed. The journey is not merely about climbing the corporate ladder but about evolving, learning, and strategically positioning oneself for opportunities. The landscape of career advancement is dynamic, influenced by various factors such as industry trends, personal aspirations, and the ever-changing demands of the job market. Understanding these elements and how they interplay is crucial for anyone looking to make significant strides in their professional life.

Career growth is a multifaceted concept that encompasses more than just promotions and salary increases. It involves personal development, acquiring new skills, and expanding one's professional network. The first step in this journey is self-assessment. Knowing your strengths, weaknesses, and areas for improvement can provide a clear roadmap for your career. This introspection helps in setting realistic and achievable goals, which are essential for long-term success. Moreover, it allows you to identify the skills and knowledge you need to acquire to stay relevant in your field.

Networking plays a pivotal role in career advancement. Building and maintaining professional relationships can open new opportunities and provide valuable insights into industry trends. Attending industry conferences, joining professional organizations, and participating in online forums are excellent ways to expand your network. These interactions can lead to mentorship opportunities, collaborations, and job offers. It's important to remember that networking is a two-way street; offering help and sharing knowledge can be as beneficial as receiving it.

Continuous learning is another cornerstone of career growth. The job market constantly evolves, and staying updated with the latest trends and technologies is crucial. Enrolling in courses, attending workshops, and obtaining certifications can enhance your skill set and make you more competitive. Additionally, seeking feedback from peers and supervisors can provide valuable insights into areas where you can improve. Embracing a growth mindset, where challenges are seen as learning opportunities, can significantly impact your career trajectory.

A detailed explanation of career growth and advancement involves understanding the various stages and strategies. The initial stage often involves gaining experience and building a solid foundation in your chosen field. This period is crucial for developing technical skills and deeply understanding industry-specific knowledge. It's also a time to explore different roles and responsibilities to identify what aligns best with your interests and strengths.

As you progress, the focus shifts towards specialization and leadership. Specializing in a particular area can make you an expert in your field, increasing your value to employers. On the other hand, leadership skills are essential for those looking to move into managerial or executive positions. These skills include effective communication, decision-making, and inspiring and motivating others. These skills can be achieved through formal training, mentorship, and practical experience.

Another critical aspect of career advancement is visibility. Being recognized for your contributions and achievements can significantly impact your career growth. This can be achieved by taking on high-visibility projects, volunteering for leadership roles, and consistently delivering high-quality work. Maintaining a professional online presence through platforms like LinkedIn can enhance your visibility and attract potential employers or collaborators.

A comprehensive review of career growth and advancement reveals several vital strategies to help individuals navigate their professional journey. One such strategy is setting SMART goals – Specific, Measurable, Achievable, Relevant, and Time-bound. These goals provide a clear direction and help in tracking progress. For instance, instead of setting a vague goal like "I want to get promoted," a SMART goal would be "I want to achieve a promotion to a senior analyst position within the next two years by completing relevant certifications and taking on additional responsibilities."

Another effective strategy is seeking mentorship. A mentor can provide guidance, share valuable insights, and help you navigate challenges. Mentorship can be formal, through structured programs, or informal, through relationships built over time. Choosing a mentor with experience in your field and whose career path aligns with your aspirations is essential.

Building a personal brand is also crucial for career advancement. Your brand is how you present yourself to the professional world and can significantly impact your career opportunities. This involves showcasing your skills, achievements, and values through various channels, such as social media, professional networks, and personal websites. A solid personal brand can differentiate you from others and make you more attractive to potential employers.

Additionally, staying adaptable and open to change is essential in today's fast-paced job market. This might involve switching industries, new roles, or even relocating for better opportunities. Being adaptable means stepping out of your comfort zone and embracing new challenges. This flexibility can lead to unexpected opportunities and accelerate your career growth.

Lastly, maintaining a healthy work-life balance is crucial for long-term career success. Burnout can hinder your productivity and overall job satisfaction. It's important to set boundaries, prioritize self-care, and make time for activities outside of work. A balanced approach ensures sustained performance and a fulfilling career.

Career growth and advancement are continuous processes that require strategic planning, constant learning, and adaptability. Individuals can navigate their professional journey more confidently and purposefully by setting clear goals, seeking mentorship, building a personal brand, and staying adaptable. The path to career advancement is not linear; it is filled with twists, turns, and occasional setbacks. However, each experience, whether positive or negative, contributes to your overall growth and resilience.

One often overlooked aspect of career growth is the importance of soft skills. While technical skills and industry knowledge are crucial, soft skills such as communication, teamwork, and emotional intelligence play a significant role in career advancement. These skills enable you to work effectively with others, navigate workplace dynamics, and lead teams successfully. Investing time in developing these skills can set you apart from your peers and enhance your professional relationships.

Communication, in particular, is a vital skill that can influence your career trajectory. Effective communication involves conveying your ideas clearly and listening actively and empathetically. Strong communication skills can help you articulate your value and build rapport with colleagues and superiors, whether presenting to a group, writing reports, or engaging in one-on-one conversations.

Emotional intelligence, or the ability to understand and manage your emotions and those of others, is another critical soft skill. High emotional intelligence can lead to better decision-making, improved conflict resolution, and stronger interpersonal relationships. It involves self-awareness, self-regulation, motivation, empathy, and social skills. Developing emotional intelligence can enhance your leadership abilities and create a positive work environment.

Another critical element in career advancement is the ability to adapt to change. The modern workplace is characterized by rapid technological advancements and shifting market demands. Being adaptable means staying open to new ideas, embracing innovation, and being willing to learn new skills. This adaptability can make you more resilient in the face of change and position you as a valuable asset to your organization.

Taking calculated risks is also an integral part of career growth. While being cautious and strategic is essential, stepping out of your comfort zone and taking on new challenges can yield significant rewards. This might involve pursuing a new role, starting a side project, or changing industries. By taking risks, you demonstrate initiative and a willingness to grow, which can be highly attractive to employers.

Moreover, seeking feedback and being open to constructive criticism can accelerate your career advancement. Feedback provides valuable insights into your performance and areas for improvement. Seeking feedback from peers, supervisors, and mentors can help you identify blind spots and make necessary adjustments. It's essential to approach feedback with a growth mindset, viewing it as an opportunity for development rather than a critique of your abilities.

In addition to seeking feedback, self-reflection is a powerful tool for career growth. Regularly reflecting on your experiences, achievements, and challenges can provide clarity and direction. This introspection allows you to assess your progress, celebrate your successes, and identify areas for improvement. Keeping a journal or engaging in mindfulness practices can facilitate this self-reflection and enhance self-awareness.

Building a solid professional reputation is another crucial aspect of career advancement. Your reputation is built on your work ethic, integrity, and the quality of your contributions. Consistently delivering high-quality work, meeting deadlines, and maintaining a positive attitude can enhance your reputation and make you a trusted and respected professional. A strong reputation can lead to new opportunities, promotions, and increased job security.

Furthermore, understanding the organizational culture and aligning yourself with its values can significantly impact your career growth. Each organization's unique culture influences decisions, how employees interact, and what behaviours are rewarded. Understanding and adapting to the organizational culture allows you to navigate workplace dynamics more effectively and position yourself for success.

Lastly, maintaining a long-term perspective is essential for sustainable career growth. While short-term goals and achievements are important, keeping an eye on your long-term aspirations and career vision is crucial. This involves regularly reassessing your goals, staying informed about industry trends, and proactively seeking new opportunities. A long-term perspective ensures that your career growth is aligned with your overall life goals and values.

Career growth and advancement are complex and multifaceted processes that require a combination of strategic planning, continuous learning, and adaptability. By focusing on self-assessment, networking, constant learning, soft skills development, adaptability, risk-taking, feedback, self-reflection, reputation building, organizational culture, and maintaining a long-term perspective, individuals can confidently navigate their professional journey and achieve their career aspirations.

Building Your Professional Brand

Building a professional brand is an essential aspect of career development. It involves creating a unique identity that distinguishes you from others in your field. This identity is built on your skills, experiences, values, and how you present yourself to the world. A solid professional brand can open doors to new opportunities, enhance your reputation, and position you as a thought leader in your industry.

The foundation of a professional brand begins with self-awareness. Understanding your strengths, weaknesses, passions, and values is crucial. This self-awareness allows you to craft an authentic brand that aligns with your identity. It's important to reflect on your career goals and the image you want to project. Are you aiming to be seen as an expert in a specific niche? Do you want to be known for your innovative thinking or leadership skills? Defining your brand's core message is the first step in building a solid professional identity.

Once you clearly understand your brand, the next step is communicating it effectively. This involves creating a consistent, compelling narrative highlighting your unique value proposition. Your narrative should be reflected in all aspects of your professional presence, from your resume and LinkedIn profile to your website and social media accounts. Consistency is vital; your brand should be recognizable and coherent across all platforms.

Networking plays a significant role in building and maintaining a professional brand. Building relationships with colleagues, mentors, and industry leaders can enhance visibility and credibility. Attending industry events, participating in online forums, and engaging with others on social media are effective ways to expand your network. Being proactive in seeking opportunities to connect with others and share your expertise is essential.

Creating and sharing content is another powerful way to build your professional brand. Writing articles, giving presentations, and participating in panel discussions can position you as a thought leader in your field. Sharing your knowledge and insights demonstrates your expertise and adds value to your audience. It's essential to be strategic in the content you create and share, ensuring that it aligns with your brand's core message and resonates with your target audience.

In addition to creating content, engaging with others' content is essential. Commenting on articles, sharing posts, and participating in discussions can help you build relationships and increase your visibility. Engaging with others meaningfully demonstrates your interest in the industry and willingness to contribute to the community.

Personal branding is not a one-time effort; it requires ongoing attention and refinement. Regularly updating your online profiles, staying current with industry trends, and continuously seeking growth opportunities are essential for maintaining a solid professional brand. It's important to be adaptable and open to feedback, as the landscape of your industry and the expectations of your audience may change over time.

A detailed topic explanation involves understanding the various components contributing to a professional brand. These components include your online presence, network, content, and personal interactions.

Your online presence is a critical aspect of your professional brand. This includes your LinkedIn profile, personal website, and social media accounts. Each platform should reflect your brand's core message and showcase your skills and experiences. A well-crafted LinkedIn profile, for example, should include a professional photo, a compelling headline, and a detailed summary of your career achievements. Your website can serve as a portfolio, highlighting your work and providing a platform for your content. Social media accounts should be used strategically to share relevant content and engage with your audience.

Personal interactions also play a significant role in building your professional brand. How you communicate with others in person and online can impact your perception. Being experienced, respectful, and authentic in your interactions is essential. Building a reliable, trustworthy, and collaborative reputation can enhance your brand and open doors to new opportunities.

A comprehensive review of the topic involves examining the various strategies and best practices for building a professional brand. One effective strategy is to identify and leverage your unique strengths and skills. This consists of conducting a self-assessment to understand what sets you apart from others in your field. Once you have identified your unique strengths, you can highlight them in your online profiles, content, and interactions.

Another best practice is to be consistent in your branding efforts. Consistency is critical to building a recognizable and coherent brand. This means ensuring that all aspects of your professional presence align with your core message. Your resume, LinkedIn profile, personal website, and social media accounts should all reflect the same narrative and showcase your unique value proposition. Consistency also extends to your interactions with others, both online and offline. Consistent communication style, tone, and messaging help reinforce your brand and build trust with your audience.

Leveraging testimonials and endorsements is another effective strategy for building a professional brand. Positive feedback from colleagues, clients, and industry leaders can enhance your credibility and provide social proof of your expertise. Including testimonials on your LinkedIn profile, personal website, and other online platforms can help to build trust and demonstrate your value to potential employers or clients.

Staying current with industry trends and developments is vital for maintaining a solid professional brand. This involves:

- Continuously seeking out opportunities for learning and growth, such as attending industry events.
- Participating in professional development courses.
- Staying informed about the latest news and trends in your field.

Being knowledgeable and up-to-date with industry developments can enhance your credibility and position you as a thought leader.

Engaging with your audience meaningfully is another best practice for building a professional brand. This involves actively participating in discussions, responding to comments and messages, and sharing valuable insights and information. Engaging with your audience demonstrates your commitment to your field and willingness to contribute to the community. It also helps to build relationships and increase your visibility.

Building a professional brand also involves being authentic to yourself. Authenticity is vital to building trust and credibility with your audience. This means being honest and transparent about your skills, experiences, and values. It also means being genuine in your interactions with others and staying true to your core message. Authenticity can help to build a strong and lasting professional brand that resonates with your audience.

In addition to these strategies, evaluating and refining your professional brand is essential. This involves periodically reviewing your online profiles, content, and interactions to ensure they align with your core message and reflect your unique value proposition. It also consists of seeking feedback from colleagues, mentors, and industry leaders to identify areas for improvement and growth. Regularly evaluating and refining your brand can help to ensure that it remains relevant and effective in achieving your career goals.

Building a professional brand is an ongoing process that requires attention, effort, and dedication. By understanding your unique strengths and skills, communicating your brand effectively, building and maintaining relationships, creating and sharing valuable content, and staying current with industry trends, you can make a solid and lasting professional brand that enhances your reputation and opens doors to new opportunities.

CHAPTER 8

ADVANCING YOUR MEDICAL CODING CAREER

Exploring Specialized Coding Roles

Specialized coding roles in the medical billing and coding field offer a unique opportunity for professionals to delve deeper into specific areas of healthcare. These roles require a thorough understanding of general coding principles and demand expertise in particular medical specialities. Mastering these specialized roles begins with a solid foundation in medical terminology, coding systems, and healthcare regulations. However, the path to specialization involves additional training, certifications, and a keen interest in the chosen field.

Medical coders who choose to specialize often find themselves working in environments that require a high level of precision and attention to detail. For instance, a coder specializing in oncology must be familiar with the intricacies of cancer diagnoses, treatments, and the specific codes associated with various types of cancer. Similarly, a cardiology coder must understand the complexities of heart-related conditions and procedures. These specialized roles enhance a coder's skill set and increase their value in the job market, often leading to higher salaries and more job opportunities.

Transitioning from a general coding role to a specialized one involves several steps. First, it's essential to identify the area of specialization that aligns with your interests and career goals. Various factors, including personal interests, job market demand, and the availability of training programs, can influence this decision. Once the area of specialization is chosen, the next step is to pursue additional education and certifications. Many professional organizations, such as the American Academy of Professional Coders (AAPC) and the American Health Information Management Association (AHIMA), offer specialized certification programs that provide the necessary training and credentials.

In addition to formal education and certifications, gaining practical experience in the chosen speciality is crucial. This can be achieved through internships, on-the-job training, or volunteering in healthcare settings focusing on the specific area of interest. Networking with professionals in the field and joining relevant professional organizations can also provide valuable insights and opportunities for career advancement. By immersing oneself in a specialized field, a coder can develop the expertise and confidence needed to excel.

Specialized coding roles are not limited to clinical settings. Many coders find opportunities in research, education, and consulting. For example, a coder with expertise in a particular speciality may work with pharmaceutical companies to ensure accurate coding of clinical trial data. Others may teach coding courses or provide consulting services to healthcare organizations looking to improve their coding practices. The versatility of specialized coding roles allows professionals to explore various career paths and find the one that best suits their skills and interests.

The demand for specialized coders is rising, driven by the increasing complexity of healthcare and the need for accurate and detailed medical records. As healthcare continues to evolve, the role of specialized coders will become even more critical. These professionals play a vital role in ensuring that medical records are accurate, complete, and compliant with regulatory requirements. Their expertise helps healthcare providers deliver better patient care, optimize reimbursement, and reduce the risk of audits and penalties.

One of the most rewarding aspects of specializing in a particular coding role is the opportunity to make a meaningful impact on patient care. By accurately coding complex medical conditions and procedures, specialized coders contribute to the overall quality of healthcare. Their work ensures that patients receive the appropriate treatments and that healthcare providers are fairly compensated. This sense of purpose and fulfilment is a significant motivator for many coders who choose to specialize.

The journey to becoming a specialized coder has its challenges. It requires a commitment to continuous learning and professional development. The healthcare industry is constantly changing, with new medical advancements, coding updates, and regulatory changes. Staying current with these changes is essential for maintaining expertise and ensuring accurate coding. Specialized coders must proactively seek educational opportunities, attend conferences, and participate in professional development activities.

In addition to technical skills, specialized coders must possess strong analytical and problem-solving abilities. They need to be able to interpret complex medical information, identify the appropriate codes, and ensure that the coding is accurate and compliant. Attention to detail is critical, as even minor errors can significantly affect patient care and reimbursement. Practical communication skills are also necessary, as specialized coders often work closely with healthcare providers, administrators, and other stakeholders.

The rewards of specializing in a particular coding role are numerous. In addition to the potential for higher salaries and job opportunities, specialized coders often enjoy greater job satisfaction and a sense of accomplishment. They become experts in their field, respected by their peers and valued by their employers. The knowledge and skills gained through specialization can also open doors to leadership and management positions, further enhancing career growth and advancement.

For those considering a specialized coding role, it's essential to take the time to research and explore the various options available. Speak with professionals in the field, attend informational sessions, and seek out mentorship opportunities. By thoroughly understanding the different specialities and the requirements for each, you can make an informed decision about the best path for your career.

Specialized coding roles offer a unique and rewarding career path for medical coders. By pursuing additional education, gaining practical experience, and staying current with industry changes, coders can transition from general coding roles to specialized positions that offer greater job satisfaction, higher earning potential, and the opportunity to impact patient care significantly. The journey to specialization is a commitment to continuous learning and professional growth, but the rewards are well worth the effort.

One of the critical benefits of specializing in a particular coding role is the ability to develop a deep understanding of a specific area of healthcare. This expertise allows coders to become valuable resources within their organizations, often as go-to experts for complex coding issues. For example, a coder specializing in orthopaedics will have an in-depth knowledge of musculoskeletal conditions, surgical procedures, and rehabilitation therapies. This specialized knowledge enhances coding accuracy, supports clinical decision-making, and improves patient outcomes.

Specialized coders also play a crucial role in ensuring healthcare regulations and standards compliance. With the ever-changing landscape of healthcare laws and policies, staying current with regulatory requirements is essential. Specialized coders must be well-versed in the specific guidelines and coding standards relevant to their expertise. This knowledge helps healthcare organizations avoid costly errors, reduce the risk of audits, and ensure proper reimbursement for services rendered.

The path to specialization often involves obtaining advanced certifications demonstrating a coder's expertise in a particular field.

These certifications, offered by reputable organizations such as AAPC and AHIMA, require rigorous training and examination. For instance, a coder interested in specializing in cardiology may pursue the Certified Cardiology Coder (CCC) credential, which validates their proficiency in coding cardiovascular procedures and diagnoses. These certifications enhance a coder's credibility and increase their marketability and career prospects.

In addition to formal certifications, specialized coders benefit from ongoing professional development and continuing education. Attending industry conferences, participating in webinars, and joining professional associations provide valuable opportunities to stay informed about the latest developments in healthcare and coding. Networking with peers and industry experts can lead to mentorship opportunities and collaborative learning experiences. By actively engaging in professional development, specialized coders can maintain their expertise and stay ahead of industry trends.

The demand for specialized coders is expected to grow as healthcare evolves and becomes more complex. Advances in medical technology, new treatments, and the increasing emphasis on value-based care require highly skilled coders with specialized knowledge. Healthcare organizations recognize the value of specialized coders in improving coding accuracy, optimizing reimbursement, and enhancing overall operational efficiency. As a result, specialized coders will likely find ample job opportunities and career advancement prospects in the coming years.

For those considering a career in specialized coding, it's essential to approach the journey with dedication and a willingness to invest in continuous learning. The rewards of specialization extend beyond financial benefits, offering a sense of professional fulfilment and the opportunity to make a meaningful impact on patient care. By choosing a speciality that aligns with their interests and career goals, coders can find a niche that challenges them and provides a sense of purpose and satisfaction.

In conclusion, specialized coding roles offer medical coders a unique and rewarding career path. By pursuing additional education, obtaining advanced certifications, and staying current with industry changes, coders can transition from general coding roles to specialized positions that offer greater job satisfaction, higher earning potential, and the opportunity to impact patient care significantly. The journey to specialization is a commitment to continuous learning and professional growth, but the rewards are well worth the effort.

Continuing Education and Certifications

Continuing education and certifications play a pivotal role in the professional development of individuals across various fields. In the ever-evolving healthcare, technology, and business landscape, staying current with the latest advancements and industry standards is crucial. For medical coders, this is particularly true. Constant changes in regulations, coding standards, and medical procedures characterize the healthcare industry. As such, medical coders must continuously learn to maintain proficiency and ensure accurate coding practices.

The journey of continuing education begins with recognizing the importance of lifelong learning. In a field as dynamic as medical coding, resting on one's laurels can lead to obsolescence. The healthcare sector demands precision, and even minor errors in coding can have significant repercussions, including financial losses and compromised patient care. Therefore, medical coders must commit to ongoing education to stay abreast of the latest coding updates, compliance requirements, and technological advancements.

Certifications testify to a coder's expertise and dedication to their profession. They provide a structured pathway for coders to deepen their knowledge and specialize in specific areas of healthcare. For instance, obtaining a Certified Professional Coder (CPC) credential from the American Academy of Professional Coders (AAPC) demonstrates a coder's proficiency in medical coding across various specialities. This certification is widely recognized and respected within the industry, enhancing a coder's credibility and career prospects.

Beyond the CPC, coders can pursue specialized certifications to further their expertise. These certifications cater to specific medical fields, such as cardiology, orthopaedics, and oncology, allowing coders to deeply understand the unique coding requirements and challenges associated with each speciality. For example, a coder specializing in cardiology may pursue the Certified Cardiology Coder (CCC) credential, which validates their proficiency in coding cardiovascular procedures and diagnoses. These specialized certifications enhance a coder's skill set and open doors to higher-paying, more fulfilling job opportunities.

Continuing education and certifications also play a crucial role in ensuring compliance with healthcare regulations. The healthcare industry is heavily regulated, with stringent guidelines governing coding practices, billing procedures, and patient privacy. Staying current with these regulations is essential to avoid costly errors, reduce the risk of audits, and ensure proper reimbursement for services rendered. By ongoing education and obtaining relevant certifications, coders can stay informed about the latest regulatory changes and ensure their coding practices align with industry standards.

The benefits of continuing education and certifications extend beyond individual coders to the organizations they work for. Healthcare providers rely on accurate coding to ensure proper billing and reimbursement, optimize revenue cycles, and maintain compliance with regulatory requirements. By investing in the professional development of their coding staff, healthcare organizations can improve coding accuracy, reduce the risk of errors, and enhance overall operational efficiency. This, in turn, leads to better financial performance and improved patient care.

For medical coders, the journey of continuing education and certification is a commitment to professional growth and excellence. It requires dedication, time, and effort, but the rewards are well worth it. By staying current with the latest industry developments, coders can enhance their skills, advance their careers, and make a meaningful impact on the healthcare industry.

Continuing education and certifications are not just about acquiring new knowledge; they are about staying relevant in a rapidly changing industry. The healthcare sector constantly evolves, with new medical procedures, technologies, and coding standards emerging regularly. Coders must continuously learn and develop professionally to keep pace with these changes. This involves attending industry conferences, participating in webinars, and joining professional associations. These activities provide valuable opportunities to stay informed about the latest developments, network with peers and industry experts, and gain insights into best practices.

Obtaining advanced certifications is a critical component of continuing education for medical coders. These certifications validate a coder's expertise in specific areas of healthcare and demonstrate their commitment to professional excellence. For example, the Certified Inpatient Coder (CIC) credential from AAPC is designed for coders who specialize in inpatient coding. This certification requires a thorough understanding of coding guidelines, medical terminology, and anatomy and the ability to code complex inpatient cases accurately. By obtaining the CIC credential, coders can enhance their credibility and career prospects and contribute to the accuracy and efficiency of inpatient coding practices.

In addition to formal certifications, continuing education involves staying current with industry trends and developments. This includes keeping up with changes in coding standards, such as updates to the International Classification of Diseases (ICD) and Current Procedural Terminology (CPT) codes. Coders must also stay informed about changes in healthcare regulations, such as updates to the Health Insurance Portability and Accountability Act (HIPAA) and the Affordable Care Act (ACA). By staying current with these changes, coders can ensure their coding practices align with industry standards and regulatory requirements.

Continuing education and certifications also provide opportunities for coders to specialize in specific areas of healthcare. Specialization allows coders to develop a deep understanding of the unique coding requirements and challenges associated with specific medical fields. For example, a coder specializing in oncology may pursue the Certified Hematology and Oncology Coder (CHONC) credential. This certification focuses on the intricacies of coding for cancer treatments, chemotherapy, and related procedures. By obtaining such specialized certifications, coders can position themselves as experts in their chosen fields, making them invaluable assets to healthcare providers who require precise and knowledgeable coding for complex medical cases.

Continuing education and certifications foster a culture of excellence and professionalism within the medical coding community. It encourages coders to strive for higher standards, stay curious, and remain committed to their professional growth. This culture of continuous improvement benefits not only the individual coders but also the broader healthcare industry. Accurate coding is essential for proper patient care, efficient billing processes, and compliance with regulatory requirements. By investing in their education and obtaining relevant certifications, coders contribute to the overall quality and integrity of the healthcare system.

Moreover, continuing education and certifications can lead to career advancement and increased earning potential for medical coders. As coders gain more knowledge and expertise, they become eligible for higher-level positions, such as coding supervisors, auditors, or educators. These roles often come with greater responsibilities and higher salaries. Additionally, specialized certifications can open doors to niche areas of coding that offer more lucrative opportunities. For example, coders with expertise in interventional radiology or surgical coding may be in high demand, commanding higher compensation for their specialized skills.

The journey of continuing education and certification has its challenges. It requires a significant investment of time, effort, and resources. Coders must balance their professional responsibilities with their educational pursuits, often studying for exams and attending training sessions outside regular working hours. However, the rewards of this investment are substantial. By staying current with industry developments and obtaining advanced certifications, coders can enhance their career prospects, contribute to the accuracy and efficiency of healthcare coding, and ultimately positively impact patient care.

The importance of continuing education and certifications for medical coders cannot be overstated in the ever-evolving healthcare landscape. These pursuits are essential for maintaining proficiency, ensuring compliance with regulatory requirements, and staying current with industry advancements. By committing to lifelong learning and obtaining relevant certifications, coders can enhance their skills, advance their careers, and contribute to the overall quality and integrity of the healthcare system. The journey of continuing education and certification is a testament to a coder's dedication to professional growth and excellence, and it is a journey that ultimately benefits both the individual coder and the broader healthcare industry.

Building a Professional Network

Networking is often considered the backbone of professional success. Building a professional network is about more than just collecting business cards or adding connections on social media platforms. It's about creating meaningful relationships that provide support, opportunities, and growth throughout your career. For beginners, networking can seem daunting, but with the right approach and mindset, it becomes an invaluable tool for career advancement.

The first step in building a professional network is understanding its importance. A strong network can open doors to new job opportunities, provide mentorship, and offer a platform for sharing knowledge and resources. It's essential to recognize that networking is a two-way street; it's not just about what you can gain but also about what you can offer others. This mutual exchange of value is what makes networking genuinely effective.

One of the most effective ways to start building a network is by attending industry events, conferences, and seminars. These gatherings provide an excellent opportunity to meet professionals in your field, learn about the latest trends and developments, and establish connections with like-minded individuals. When attending these events, it's crucial to be prepared. Have a clear understanding of your goals, be ready to introduce yourself confidently, and have a few conversation starters in mind. Remember, the goal is to build genuine relationships, so focus on listening and engaging in meaningful conversations rather than just promoting yourself.

Another valuable strategy for building a professional network is leveraging online platforms. LinkedIn, for example, is a powerful tool for connecting with professionals across various industries. Create a compelling profile that highlights your skills, experiences, and achievements. Join relevant groups and participate in discussions to showcase your expertise and connect with others who share your interests. Additionally, don't hesitate to reach out to individuals you admire or those who work in companies you're interested in. A well-crafted message expressing your interest and admiration can go a long way in establishing a connection.

Mentorship is another critical aspect of networking. Finding a mentor who can guide you, provide insights, and help you navigate your career path can be incredibly beneficial. Look for individuals who have succeeded in your field and reach out to them with a genuine request for mentorship. Respect their time and clarify what you hope to gain from the relationship. A good mentor can offer invaluable advice, introduce you to their network, and help you avoid common pitfalls in your career.

Networking is not limited to formal events or online platforms. Everyday interactions also provide opportunities to build your network. Engage with colleagues, participate in team projects, and use collaboration opportunities. Building strong relationships within your workplace can lead to new opportunities and provide a support system that can be invaluable throughout your career.

Volunteering is another excellent way to expand your network. You can meet individuals who share your values and interests by offering your time and skills to causes you care about. Volunteering provides opportunities to develop new skills, gain experience, and demonstrate your commitment to making a positive impact. These experiences can be valuable additions to your resume and help you stand out in the job market.

Building a professional network requires time, effort, and a genuine interest in connecting with others. Patience and persistence are essential as meaningful relationships develop over time. Regularly follow up with your connections, offer assistance when needed, and stay engaged with your network. By nurturing these relationships, you can create a solid and supportive network that will benefit you throughout your career.

A detailed explanation of building a professional network involves understanding the various components and strategies contributing to effective networking. One of the critical elements is the ability to communicate effectively. Good communication skills are essential for making a positive impression and building rapport. This includes being able to articulate your thoughts clearly, listening actively, and showing genuine interest in the conversations you have.

Another critical aspect of networking is the ability to identify and seize opportunities. This requires being proactive and staying informed about industry events, job openings, and other possible opportunities. It's also important to be open to new experiences and willing to step out of your comfort zone. By being proactive and open-minded, you can take advantage of opportunities to help you grow your network and advance your career.

Building a professional network also involves being strategic about the connections you make. It's essential to focus on quality rather than quantity. Instead of connecting with as many people as possible, focus on building meaningful relationships with individuals who can provide value and support. This includes seeking mentors, industry leaders, and peers who share your interests and goals.

Another critical strategy for building a professional network is to provide value to others. This can be done by sharing your knowledge and expertise, offering assistance, and being a reliable and supportive connection. By providing value to others, you can build a reputation as a valuable and trustworthy professional, which can help you attract and retain meaningful connections.

It's also important to stay engaged with your network. This involves:

- Regularly following up with your connections.
- Staying informed about their achievements and challenges.
- Offering your support when needed.
-

By staying engaged and maintaining regular communication with your network, you demonstrate your commitment to the relationships you've built, which can lead to deeper and more meaningful connections over time.

Developing Leadership Skills

Leadership is a multifaceted skill beyond simply managing a team or making decisions. It encompasses a range of abilities, including communication, empathy, strategic thinking, and the capacity to inspire and motivate others. Developing leadership skills is essential for anyone aspiring to advance in their career, as it enables individuals to effectively guide their teams, drive organizational success, and foster a positive work environment. Becoming a proficient leader involves continuous learning, self-reflection, and applying various techniques and strategies practically.

One of the foundational aspects of leadership is self-awareness. Understanding your strengths, weaknesses, values, and motivations allows you to lead authentically and honestly. Self-aware leaders are better equipped to make informed decisions, manage their emotions, and build trust with their team members. To enhance self-awareness, consider seeking feedback from colleagues, mentors, and peers. Reflect on your experiences and identify areas for improvement. Regular self-assessment can help you stay aligned with your goals and values, making you a more effective leader.

Effective communication is another critical component of leadership. Leaders must convey their vision, expectations, and feedback clearly and persuasively. This involves not only speaking but also listening actively and empathetically. Active listening fosters a culture of openness and respect, where team members feel valued and heard.

To improve your communication skills, practice active listening, ask open-ended questions, and be mindful of non-verbal cues. Additionally, tailor your communication style to suit your audience's needs and preferences, whether through written reports, presentations, or one-on-one conversations.

Empathy is a powerful tool in a leader's arsenal. By understanding and addressing the emotions and perspectives of others, leaders can build strong, supportive relationships with their team members. Empathetic leaders are likelier to create a positive work environment where employees feel motivated and engaged. To cultivate empathy, understand your team members' challenges and concerns. Show genuine interest in their well-being and provide support when needed. Empathy also involves recognizing and appreciating your team's diverse backgrounds and experiences, fostering an inclusive and collaborative culture.

Strategic thinking is essential for effective leadership. Leaders must be able to anticipate future trends, identify opportunities, and develop long-term plans that align with organizational goals. Strategic thinking involves analyzing complex situations, considering multiple perspectives, and making informed decisions based on data and insights. To enhance your strategic thinking skills, stay informed about industry trends, continuously learn, and seek diverse viewpoints. Collaborate with colleagues and mentors to brainstorm ideas and develop innovative solutions.

Inspiring and motivating others is a hallmark of outstanding leadership. Leaders who articulate a compelling vision and rally their team around a common goal are more likely to succeed. Inspiration comes from leading by example, demonstrating passion and commitment, and recognizing and celebrating your team's achievements. To inspire and motivate your team, communicate a clear and compelling vision, set achievable goals, and provide regular feedback and recognition. Encourage a growth mindset where team members feel empowered to take risks, learn from failures, and continuously improve.

Leadership also involves making tough decisions and taking responsibility for the outcomes. Decisive leaders can weigh the pros and cons of various options, consider the impact on stakeholders, and make informed choices that align with organizational values and goals. To improve your decision-making skills, gather relevant information, consult with trusted advisors, and consider the long-term implications of your choices. Be transparent about your decision-making process and be willing to take accountability for the results.

Building and leading high-performing teams is another crucial aspect of leadership. Influential leaders understand the importance of collaboration, trust, and mutual respect within a team. They create an environment where team members feel empowered to contribute their unique skills and perspectives. To build a high-performing team, foster a culture of trust and collaboration. Encourage open communication, provide opportunities for professional development, and recognize and reward the contributions of your team members. Additionally, proactively address conflicts and challenges and provide support and guidance to help your team navigate obstacles.

Leadership development is an ongoing process that requires continuous learning and growth. Seek opportunities for professional development, such as leadership training programs, workshops, and conferences. Engage with mentors and peers who can provide valuable insights and guidance. Reflect on your experiences and learn from both successes and failures. By committing to continuous improvement, you can develop the skills and qualities needed to be an effective and inspiring leader.

In summary, developing leadership skills involves a combination of self-awareness, effective communication, empathy, strategic thinking, and the ability to inspire and motivate others. It requires a commitment to continuous learning and growth and the willingness to take on challenges and make tough decisions. Focusing on these critical areas can enhance your leadership abilities and drive success for yourself and your team.

Leadership is not a one-size-fits-all concept; it varies depending on the context, the team, and the individual leader's style. Some leaders may excel in strategic thinking, while others may be more adept at building strong relationships and fostering collaboration and trust. The most effective leaders can adapt their style to meet their team's needs and the situation's demands. This adaptability requires a deep understanding of various leadership approaches and the ability to apply them as needed.

Work-Life Balance for Coding Professionals

Balancing work and personal life is a challenge that many coding professionals face. The nature of the job often demands long hours, intense focus, and continuous learning, which can easily spill over into personal time. This imbalance can lead to burnout, decreased productivity, and strained relationships. Understanding the importance of work-life balance and implementing strategies to achieve it is crucial for maintaining both professional success and personal well-being.

Coding professionals often find themselves in a cycle of constant work driven by deadlines, the need to stay updated with the latest technologies, and the intrinsic passion for coding. This dedication, while commendable, can lead to neglecting personal life, hobbies, and even health. The pressure to perform and the competitive nature of the tech industry can exacerbate this issue, making it seem like there is never enough time to relax or disconnect from work.

One of the critical aspects of achieving work-life balance is setting clear boundaries. This involves defining and sticking to specific work hours as much as possible. Communicating these boundaries to colleagues and supervisors is essential to ensure they are respected. Creating a dedicated workspace at home can help mentally separate work from personal life. When the workday ends, physically leaving the workspace can signal the end of work time and the beginning of personal time.

Another critical strategy is prioritizing tasks. Not all tasks are created equal, and understanding which ones are most critical can help manage time more effectively. Using tools like to-do lists, project management software, and time-tracking apps can aid in organizing tasks and ensuring that critical deadlines are met without sacrificing personal time. It's also beneficial to break down larger tasks into smaller, manageable chunks, making them less overwhelming and more accessible within the allotted work hours.

Taking regular breaks is another crucial element in maintaining a work-life balance. Continuous work without breaks can lead to mental fatigue and decreased productivity. Short breaks throughout the day help recharge and maintain focus. Also, longer breaks, such as walking or engaging in a hobby, can provide a much-needed mental reset. Taking vacations and time off is essential to disconnect from work and recharge fully.

Physical health plays a significant role in achieving work-life balance. Regular exercise, a healthy diet, and adequate sleep are essential for maintaining energy levels and overall well-being. Coding professionals often spend long hours in front of a computer, leading to physical strain and health issues. Incorporating physical activity into the daily routine, such as stretching, walking, or even short workout sessions, can help mitigate these effects and improve overall health.

Mental health is equally important. The stress and pressure of the job can take a toll on mental well-being. Mindfulness, meditation, or other relaxation techniques can help manage stress and maintain a positive mindset. It's also essential to seek support when needed, whether talking to a friend, family member, or a mental health professional. Building a support network can provide a sense of community and help navigate balancing work and personal life challenges.

Engaging in hobbies and activities outside work is another effective way to achieve work-life balance. Hobbies provide a creative outlet and a way to unwind and relax.

 Whether reading, painting, playing a musical instrument, or any other activity, dedicating time to hobbies can help maintain a healthy balance between work and personal life. Spending quality time with family and friends is also beneficial, as social connections are essential for overall well-being.

Incorporating these strategies into daily life requires commitment and consistency. It's essential to regularly assess and adjust the approach to work-life balance based on changing circumstances and needs. Flexibility is critical, as what works at one point may need to be adjusted as personal and professional situations evolve. It's also important to recognize that achieving work-life balance is an ongoing process, not a one-time goal.

The benefits of achieving work-life balance are numerous. It leads to increased productivity, as a well-rested and mentally healthy individual is more capable of performing at their best. It also reduces the risk of burnout, which can negatively affect personal and professional life. Also, maintaining a healthy work-life balance can lead to improved relationships, as more time and energy are needed to dedicate to family and friends.

Achieving a work-life balance for coding professionals can also increase job satisfaction. When personal and professional lives are in harmony, there is a greater sense of fulfillment and purpose. This can lead to increased motivation and a more positive outlook on work. It also allows for personal growth and development, as there is time to pursue interests and hobbies outside work.

In conclusion, work-life balance is essential for coding professionals to maintain professional success and personal well-being. Coding professionals can balance work and personal life by setting clear boundaries, prioritizing tasks, taking regular breaks, maintaining physical and mental health, and engaging in hobbies and activities outside work. This balance leads to increased productivity, reduced risk of burnout, improved relationships, and greater job satisfaction.

CHAPTER 9

HEALTHCARE TECHNOLOGY AND INNOVATIONS

Electronic Health Records (EHR) Systems

Electronic Health Records (EHR) systems have revolutionized the healthcare industry, transforming how patient information is stored, accessed, and managed. These digital records replace traditional paper-based systems, offering a more efficient and streamlined approach to handling medical data. The adoption of EHR systems has been driven by the need for improved patient care, enhanced data accuracy, and better coordination among healthcare providers. By digitizing patient records, EHR systems facilitate real-time access to critical information, enabling healthcare professionals to make informed decisions quickly and accurately.

The implementation of EHR systems has brought about significant changes in the way healthcare is delivered. One of the primary benefits is the ability to access patient information from anywhere at any time. This accessibility is particularly crucial in emergency situations where timely access to medical history can be life-saving. EHR systems also support the integration of various healthcare services, allowing for seamless communication and collaboration among different providers. This integration ensures that all relevant information is available to the entire care team, reducing the risk of errors and improving overall patient outcomes.

Another key advantage of EHR systems is the enhancement of data accuracy and completeness. Traditional paper records are prone to errors, such as illegible handwriting, missing information, and duplication. EHR systems eliminate these issues by providing a standardized format for data entry, ensuring that all necessary information is captured accurately. Additionally, EHR systems often include built-in checks and alerts to prevent common errors, such as drug interactions or incorrect dosages. This level of accuracy is essential for delivering safe and effective patient care.

EHR systems also play a crucial role in improving the efficiency of healthcare operations. By automating routine tasks, such as appointment scheduling, billing, and prescription refills, EHR systems free up valuable time for healthcare professionals to focus on patient care. This automation reduces administrative burdens and streamlines workflows, leading to increased productivity and cost savings. Furthermore, EHR systems enable better resource management by providing insights into patient demographics, treatment patterns, and resource utilization. These insights can inform strategic planning and decision-making, ultimately enhancing the quality of care provided.

The detailed explanation of EHR systems delves into their core functionalities and the impact they have on healthcare delivery. At the heart of EHR systems is the electronic storage of patient information, which includes medical history, diagnoses, medications, immunization records, lab results, and imaging reports. This comprehensive repository of data provides a holistic view of the patient's health, enabling healthcare providers to deliver personalized and coordinated care. EHR systems also support the documentation of clinical encounters, allowing for accurate and timely recording of patient interactions.

One of the critical features of EHR systems is interoperability, which refers to the ability to exchange and use information across different healthcare settings. Interoperability ensures that patient data can be shared seamlessly among hospitals, clinics, laboratories, and other healthcare entities. This capability is vital for continuity of care, as it allows for the transfer of essential information when patients move between different providers or levels of care.

EHR systems achieve interoperability through standardized data formats and communication protocols, such as Health Level Seven (HL7) and Fast Healthcare Interoperability Resources (FHIR).

EHR systems also incorporate decision support tools that assist healthcare providers in making evidence-based decisions. These tools include clinical guidelines, diagnostic algorithms, and predictive analytics, which provide real-time recommendations based on the patient's data. Decision support tools enhance the quality of care by ensuring that providers have access to the latest medical knowledge and best practices. Additionally, EHR systems often feature patient portals, which empower patients to take an active role in their healthcare. Through these portals, patients can access their medical records, schedule appointments, request prescription refills, and communicate with their providers.

The comprehensive review of EHR systems highlights their transformative impact on healthcare delivery. One of the most significant benefits is the improvement in patient safety. EHR systems reduce the risk of medical errors by providing accurate and up-to-date information, alerting providers to potential issues, and ensuring that all relevant data is available at the point of care. For example, EHR systems can flag potential drug interactions or allergies, preventing adverse reactions and ensuring that patients receive appropriate treatments. This level of safety is particularly important in complex cases where multiple providers are involved in the patient's care.

EHR systems also enhance the quality of care by facilitating evidence-based practice. By providing access to clinical guidelines and decision support tools, EHR systems ensure that healthcare providers can make informed decisions based on the latest medical research. This evidence-based approach leads to better patient outcomes and more consistent care across different providers and settings. Additionally, EHR systems support population health management by enabling the analysis of large datasets to identify trends, track outcomes, and develop targeted interventions. This capability is essential for addressing public health challenges and improving the overall health of communities.

Another critical aspect of EHR systems is their role in enhancing patient engagement. By providing patients with access to their medical records and enabling them to participate in their care, EHR systems empower individuals to take control of their health. Patient portals, for example, allow patients to view test results, track their progress, and communicate directly with their healthcare providers. This transparency fosters a sense of ownership and responsibility, encouraging patients to adhere to treatment plans and make informed decisions about their health. Additionally, EHR systems can send automated reminders for appointments, medication refills, and preventive screenings, helping patients stay on top of their healthcare needs.

Computer-Assisted Coding and Auditing

Computer-assisted coding (CAC) and auditing have revolutionized the healthcare industry, offering a blend of technology and expertise to streamline processes and enhance accuracy. These systems leverage advanced algorithms to analyze clinical documentation and assign appropriate medical codes, which are essential for billing, reimbursement, and data analysis. The integration of CAC and auditing tools into healthcare practices has significantly reduced the burden on human coders, minimized errors, and improved compliance with regulatory standards.

The journey of CAC begins with the extraction of relevant information from electronic health records (EHRs). This information includes patient demographics, clinical notes, lab results, and diagnostic imaging reports. The CAC system then processes this data using natural language processing (NLP) and other sophisticated techniques to identify key terms and phrases that correspond to specific medical codes. By automating this process, CAC systems can quickly and accurately assign codes, reducing the time and effort required by human coders.

One of the primary benefits of CAC is its ability to enhance coding accuracy. Human coders, despite their expertise, are prone to errors due to the sheer volume and complexity of medical documentation. CAC systems, on the other hand, can analyze vast amounts of data with precision, ensuring that the correct codes are assigned based on the clinical documentation. This accuracy is crucial for proper billing and reimbursement, as incorrect codes can lead to denied claims and financial losses for healthcare providers.

In addition to improving accuracy, CAC systems also increase efficiency. Traditional coding methods can be time-consuming, with coders spending hours sifting through documentation to identify relevant information. CAC systems can perform this task in a fraction of the time, allowing coders to focus on more complex cases that require human judgment. This increased efficiency not only speeds up the coding process but also reduces the workload on coders, preventing burnout and improving job satisfaction.

Auditing is another critical aspect of the healthcare industry that has been transformed by technology. Computer-assisted auditing tools are designed to review coded data for accuracy and compliance with regulatory standards. These tools can identify discrepancies, such as incorrect codes or missing documentation, and flag them for further review. By automating the auditing process, healthcare organizations can ensure that their coding practices are compliant with industry standards and reduce the risk of financial penalties.

The implementation of CAC and auditing systems requires careful planning and consideration. Healthcare organizations must invest in the right technology and ensure that their staff is adequately trained to use these tools effectively. This includes understanding the capabilities and limitations of CAC systems, as well as knowing when to rely on human judgment for complex cases. Additionally, organizations must establish clear protocols for auditing and addressing discrepancies identified by the system.

Despite the numerous benefits, there are challenges associated with the adoption of CAC and auditing tools. One of the primary concerns is the initial cost of implementation, which includes purchasing the software, training staff, and integrating the system with existing EHRs. However, many organizations find that the long-term benefits, such as increased accuracy and efficiency, outweigh these initial expenses.

Another challenge is ensuring the security and privacy of patient data. CAC and auditing systems must comply with stringent regulations to protect sensitive information. This involves implementing robust security measures, such as encryption and access controls, to prevent unauthorized access and data breaches. Healthcare organizations must also educate their staff on best practices for data security and privacy to mitigate risks.

The transition to CAC and auditing tools can also be met with resistance from staff who are accustomed to traditional coding and auditing methods. This resistance can be overcome through comprehensive training programs that demonstrate the benefits of these systems and provide hands-on experience with the new technology. Additionally, involving staff in the selection and implementation process can help address concerns and foster a sense of ownership and acceptance.

The integration of CAC and auditing tools into healthcare practices has the potential to revolutionize the industry. By automating the coding and auditing processes, these systems can enhance accuracy, increase efficiency, and improve compliance with regulatory standards. This not only benefits healthcare providers by reducing the risk of financial penalties but also ensures that patients receive accurate billing and reimbursement for their care.

As technology continues to advance, CAC and auditing systems are likely to evolve, incorporating new features and capabilities that further enhance their value. For example, the integration of machine learning algorithms can provide even more sophisticated analysis and decision support, improving the accuracy and efficiency of coding and auditing processes. Additionally, advancements in interoperability standards will facilitate greater data sharing and collaboration across the healthcare ecosystem.

The future of CAC and auditing holds great promise for transforming healthcare delivery and improving patient outcomes. By embracing these digital tools and addressing the challenges associated with their implementation, healthcare organizations can unlock the full potential of CAC and auditing systems and pave the way for a more efficient, effective, and patient-centered healthcare system.

Artificial Intelligence in Medical Coding

The integration of artificial intelligence (AI) into medical coding represents a significant advancement in the healthcare industry. Medical coding, a critical process that involves translating healthcare diagnoses, procedures, medical services, and equipment into universal medical alphanumeric codes, has traditionally been a labor-intensive and error-prone task. The advent of AI technologies promises to revolutionize this field by enhancing accuracy, efficiency, and consistency. AI systems can analyze vast amounts of data quickly, identify patterns, and make predictions, which can significantly reduce the burden on human coders and improve the overall quality of medical coding.

AI-driven medical coding systems utilize machine learning algorithms to learn from vast datasets of medical records. These systems can automatically extract relevant information from clinical documentation and assign appropriate codes. This automation not only speeds up the coding process but also minimizes the risk of human error. For instance, natural language processing (NLP), a subset of AI, enables machines to understand and interpret human language, making it possible to accurately extract and code information from unstructured clinical notes. This capability is particularly valuable in handling the complexity and variability of medical language.

Moreover, AI can assist in ensuring compliance with coding standards and regulations. By continuously learning from new data and updates in coding guidelines, AI systems can stay current with the latest changes in medical coding practices. This dynamic adaptability is crucial in a field where regulations and standards are frequently updated. Additionally, AI can provide real-time feedback to human coders, highlighting potential errors or discrepancies and suggesting corrections. This collaborative approach not only enhances the accuracy of coding but also serves as a valuable educational tool for coders, helping them improve their skills and knowledge over time.

The implementation of AI in medical coding also has significant implications for healthcare providers and patients. For healthcare providers, AI-driven coding systems can lead to substantial cost savings by reducing the need for extensive manual coding efforts and minimizing the risk of costly coding errors. Accurate coding is essential for proper billing and reimbursement, and errors in coding can result in denied claims or financial losses. By improving the accuracy and efficiency of coding, AI can help healthcare providers optimize their revenue cycle management and ensure timely and accurate reimbursement for services rendered.

For patients, the benefits of AI in medical coding are equally compelling. Accurate coding is essential for maintaining comprehensive and accurate medical records, which are crucial for effective patient care. Errors in coding can lead to incorrect diagnoses, inappropriate treatments, and potential harm to patients.

By enhancing the accuracy of coding, AI can contribute to better patient outcomes and improved quality of care. Additionally, AI-driven coding systems can help identify patterns and trends in patient data, enabling healthcare providers to make more informed decisions and deliver personalized care.

Despite the numerous advantages of AI in medical coding, there are also challenges and considerations that need to be addressed. One of the primary concerns is the potential for bias in AI algorithms. If the training data used to develop AI systems is biased or unrepresentative, the resulting algorithms may perpetuate or even exacerbate existing disparities in healthcare. It is essential to ensure that AI systems are trained on diverse and representative datasets to minimize the risk of bias and ensure equitable outcomes for all patients.

Another challenge is the need for robust data privacy and security measures. Medical coding involves handling sensitive patient information, and the use of AI systems raises concerns about data privacy and security. Healthcare organizations must implement stringent measures to protect patient data and ensure compliance with regulations such as the Health Insurance Portability and Accountability Act (HIPAA). Additionally, there is a need for transparency and explainability in AI algorithms. Healthcare providers and coders must understand how AI systems arrive at their coding decisions to ensure accountability and trust in the technology.

The integration of AI in medical coding also requires a shift in the roles and responsibilities of human coders. While AI can automate many aspects of the coding process, human expertise remains essential for handling complex cases, making nuanced judgments, and ensuring the overall quality of coding. Human coders will need to adapt to new workflows and collaborate with AI systems, leveraging their expertise to validate and refine AI-generated codes. This collaboration between humans and machines can lead to a more efficient and accurate coding process, ultimately benefiting the entire healthcare ecosystem.

In conclusion, the integration of AI into medical coding holds great promise for transforming the healthcare industry. By enhancing the accuracy, efficiency, and consistency of coding, AI can reduce the burden on human coders, improve compliance with coding standards, and optimize revenue cycle management for healthcare providers. Patients stand to benefit from more accurate medical records, better patient outcomes, and personalized care. However, it is crucial to address challenges related to bias, data privacy, and the evolving role of human coders to fully realize the potential of AI in medical coding. As the technology continues to evolve, ongoing collaboration between AI developers, healthcare providers, and policymakers will be essential to ensure that AI-driven medical coding systems are effective, equitable, and trustworthy.

Cybersecurity and Data Privacy

In the digital age, cybersecurity and data privacy have become paramount concerns for individuals and organizations alike. The rapid advancement of technology has brought about unprecedented convenience and connectivity, but it has also introduced new vulnerabilities and threats. Cybersecurity refers to the measures and practices designed to protect systems, networks, and data from cyberattacks, while data privacy focuses on safeguarding personal information from unauthorized access and misuse. Understanding these concepts is crucial for navigating the modern digital landscape safely and responsibly.

The importance of cybersecurity cannot be overstated. Cyberattacks can lead to significant financial losses, reputational damage, and legal repercussions. From phishing scams and ransomware attacks to data breaches and identity theft, the range of cyber threats is vast and ever-evolving. Hackers and cybercriminals are constantly devising new methods to exploit vulnerabilities, making it essential for individuals and organizations to stay vigilant and proactive in their cybersecurity efforts.

Data privacy, on the other hand, is concerned with the proper handling of personal information. This includes how data is collected, stored, shared, and used. With the proliferation of online services and social media platforms, vast amounts of personal data are being generated and shared daily. Ensuring that this data is protected from unauthorized access and misuse is critical for maintaining trust and safeguarding individual privacy rights.

One of the fundamental principles of cybersecurity is the implementation of strong passwords and authentication methods. Passwords should be complex, unique, and regularly updated to minimize the risk of unauthorized access. Multi-factor authentication (MFA) adds an extra layer of security by requiring users to provide additional verification, such as a fingerprint or a one-time code sent to their mobile device. This makes it significantly more difficult for attackers to gain access to sensitive information.

Another key aspect of cybersecurity is the use of encryption. Encryption involves converting data into a coded format that can only be deciphered by authorized parties. This ensures that even if data is intercepted during transmission, it remains unreadable to unauthorized individuals. Encryption is widely used in various applications, from securing online transactions to protecting sensitive communications.

Regular software updates and patches are also crucial for maintaining cybersecurity. Software developers frequently release updates to address security vulnerabilities and improve functionality. Failing to install these updates can leave systems exposed to known threats. It is essential to keep all software, including operating systems, applications, and antivirus programs, up to date to ensure maximum protection.

In addition to technical measures, cybersecurity also involves raising awareness and educating users about potential threats. Phishing attacks, for example, often rely on social engineering techniques to trick individuals into revealing sensitive information. By educating users about the signs of phishing attempts and encouraging them to exercise caution when clicking on links or downloading attachments, organizations can significantly reduce the risk of successful attacks.

Data privacy, meanwhile, requires a comprehensive approach to managing personal information. Organizations must implement robust data protection policies and practices to ensure that personal data is collected, stored, and used in compliance with relevant regulations. This includes obtaining explicit consent from individuals before collecting their data, providing clear information about how their data will be used, and offering options for individuals to control their data.

One of the key regulations governing data privacy is the General Data Protection Regulation (GDPR) in the European Union. The GDPR sets strict guidelines for the collection, processing, and storage of personal data, and imposes significant penalties for non-compliance. Organizations operating within the EU or handling the data of EU citizens must adhere to these regulations to avoid legal repercussions and maintain trust with their customers.

Another important aspect of data privacy is data minimization. This principle involves collecting only the minimum amount of personal data necessary for a specific purpose and retaining it only for as long as needed. By minimizing the amount of data collected and stored, organizations can reduce the risk of data breaches and ensure that they are handling personal information responsibly.

Data anonymization and pseudonymization are additional techniques used to protect privacy. Anonymization involves removing or altering personal identifiers from data sets so that individuals cannot be identified. Pseudonymization, on the other hand, replaces personal identifiers with pseudonyms, allowing data to be used for analysis without revealing the identities of individuals. These techniques help organizations balance the need for data analysis with the requirement to protect individual privacy.

The rise of cloud computing has also introduced new challenges and opportunities for cybersecurity and data privacy. Cloud services offer scalability, flexibility, and cost savings, but they also require careful consideration of security and privacy risks. Organizations must ensure that their cloud service providers implement robust security measures and comply with relevant data protection regulations. This includes encrypting data stored in the cloud, regularly auditing security practices, and establishing clear data ownership and access controls.

In the context of cybersecurity and data privacy, it is also important to consider the role of emerging technologies such as artificial intelligence (AI) and the Internet of Things (IoT). AI can enhance cybersecurity by identifying and responding to threats more quickly and accurately than traditional methods. However, it also introduces new risks, such as the potential for AI systems to be manipulated or used for malicious purposes. Similarly, IoT devices, which are often connected to the internet and collect vast amounts of data, present unique security challenges. Many IoT devices lack robust security features, making them vulnerable to attacks. Ensuring the security of these devices requires a multi-faceted approach, including secure device design, regular firmware updates, and network segmentation to isolate IoT devices from critical systems.

The human element remains one of the most significant factors in cybersecurity and data privacy. Human error, negligence, or malicious intent can undermine even the most sophisticated security measures. Insider threats, whether intentional or accidental, pose a significant risk to organizations. Implementing comprehensive security training programs and fostering a culture of security awareness can help mitigate these risks. Employees should be educated on best practices, such as recognizing phishing attempts, securely handling sensitive information, and reporting suspicious activities.

Incident response planning is another critical component of cybersecurity. Despite best efforts, breaches and attacks can still occur. Having a well-defined incident response plan ensures that organizations can quickly and effectively respond to security incidents, minimizing damage and facilitating recovery. This plan should include procedures for identifying and containing the breach, notifying affected parties, and conducting a thorough investigation to prevent future incidents.

Collaboration and information sharing are also vital in the fight against cyber threats. Governments, private sector organizations, and cybersecurity professionals must work together to share threat intelligence, develop best practices, and coordinate responses to emerging threats. Public-private partnerships and industry-specific information sharing and analysis centers (ISACs) play a crucial role in enhancing collective cybersecurity resilience.

The legal and regulatory landscape surrounding cybersecurity and data privacy is continually evolving. Governments worldwide are enacting new laws and regulations to address the growing threat of cybercrime and protect personal data. Organizations must stay informed about these developments and ensure compliance with applicable laws. This includes conducting regular audits, updating policies and procedures, and engaging with legal and regulatory experts to navigate the complex landscape.

Ethical considerations also play a significant role in cybersecurity and data privacy. Organizations must balance the need for security with respect for individual privacy rights. This involves making ethical decisions about data collection, usage, and sharing. Transparency and accountability are key principles in building trust with customers and stakeholders. Organizations should be open about their data practices and take responsibility for protecting personal information.

The future of cybersecurity and data privacy will be shaped by ongoing technological advancements and evolving threat landscapes. Quantum computing, for example, has the potential to revolutionize encryption methods, but it also poses new challenges for current cryptographic techniques. Staying ahead of these developments requires continuous research, innovation, and adaptation.

In conclusion, cybersecurity and data privacy are critical components of the modern digital landscape. Protecting systems, networks, and personal information from cyber threats requires a comprehensive and proactive approach. This includes implementing strong technical measures, fostering a culture of security awareness, staying informed about legal and regulatory developments, and making ethical decisions about data handling. By prioritizing cybersecurity and data privacy, individuals and organizations can navigate the digital world safely and responsibly, ensuring the protection of sensitive information and maintaining trust in the digital ecosystem.

Future Trends and Emerging Technologies

The rapid pace of technological advancement continues to shape the future in ways that were once the realm of science fiction. As we stand on the cusp of a new era, several trends and emerging technologies promise to revolutionize various aspects of our lives. From the way we communicate and work to how we manage our health and interact with the world around us, these innovations are set to redefine the boundaries of possibility.

One of the most significant trends is the increasing integration of technology into our daily lives through the Internet of Things (IoT). This network of interconnected devices, ranging from smart home appliances to wearable health monitors, is creating a seamless digital ecosystem. IoT devices collect and share data, enabling more efficient and personalized experiences. For instance, smart thermostats can learn your preferences and adjust the temperature accordingly, while wearable fitness trackers provide real-time health insights. The potential applications of IoT are vast, spanning industries such as healthcare, agriculture, and transportation.

Another transformative trend is the rise of 5G technology. This next-generation wireless network promises faster speeds, lower latency, and greater connectivity. With 5G, downloading a high-definition movie could take mere seconds, and remote surgeries could become a reality. The enhanced capabilities of 5G will also drive the development of smart cities, where everything from traffic lights to waste management systems is interconnected and optimized for efficiency. The deployment of 5G networks is expected to unlock new possibilities for innovation and economic growth.

In the realm of healthcare, advancements in biotechnology and personalized medicine are paving the way for more effective treatments and improved patient outcomes. Gene editing technologies, such as CRISPR, hold the potential to cure genetic disorders by precisely altering DNA sequences. Personalized medicine, which tailors treatments based on an individual's genetic makeup, is becoming increasingly feasible with advancements in genomics and data analytics. These innovations are not only enhancing our understanding of diseases but also enabling the development of targeted therapies that minimize side effects and maximize efficacy.

The field of renewable energy is also witnessing significant breakthroughs. As the world grapples with the challenges of climate change, the transition to sustainable energy sources is more critical than ever. Innovations in solar and wind energy, along with advancements in energy storage technologies, are making renewable energy more accessible and cost-effective. For example, the development of more efficient solar panels and wind turbines is increasing the viability of these energy sources. Additionally, improvements in battery technology are addressing the intermittency issues associated with renewable energy, enabling more reliable and consistent power supply.

In the realm of transportation, autonomous vehicles are poised to revolutionize the way we travel. Self-driving cars, trucks, and drones are being developed and tested by various companies, with the promise of safer and more efficient transportation systems. Autonomous vehicles have the potential to reduce traffic accidents, lower emissions, and improve mobility for individuals with disabilities. The widespread adoption of autonomous vehicles will also have far-reaching implications for urban planning, as cities may need to adapt their infrastructure to accommodate these new modes of transportation.

The concept of the metaverse is another emerging trend that is capturing the imagination of technologists and futurists alike. The metaverse is a virtual, interconnected universe where people can interact, work, and play in immersive digital environments. Powered by advancements in virtual reality (VR) and augmented reality (AR), the metaverse offers new possibilities for social interaction, entertainment, and commerce. Imagine attending a virtual concert with friends from around the world or collaborating on a project in a digital workspace that feels as real as a physical office. The metaverse has the potential to blur the lines between the physical and digital worlds, creating new opportunities for connection and creativity.

Blockchain technology, best known for underpinning cryptocurrencies like Bitcoin, is also gaining traction in various industries. Beyond digital currencies, blockchain offers a decentralized and secure way to record transactions and manage data. This technology has the potential to transform sectors such as finance, supply chain management, and healthcare by enhancing transparency, reducing fraud, and streamlining processes. For example, blockchain can be used to track the provenance of goods, ensuring that products are ethically sourced and authentic. In healthcare, blockchain can provide a secure and interoperable platform for managing patient records, improving data sharing and collaboration among healthcare providers.

Quantum computing is another frontier that holds immense promise. Unlike classical computers, which use bits to process information, quantum computers use quantum bits or qubits. This allows them to perform complex calculations at unprecedented speeds. While still in the experimental stage, quantum computing has the potential to revolutionize fields such as cryptography, materials science, and drug discovery. For instance, quantum computers could break current encryption methods, necessitating the development of new cryptographic techniques. In materials science, quantum simulations could lead to the discovery of new materials with unique properties, while in drug discovery, quantum computing could accelerate the identification of potential drug candidates.

The convergence of these emerging technologies is creating a landscape of unprecedented innovation and opportunity. However, it also raises important ethical and societal questions. As technology becomes more integrated into our lives, issues such as data privacy, security, and digital equity become increasingly critical. Ensuring that the benefits of these advancements are equitably distributed and that individuals' rights are protected will be paramount. Policymakers, technologists, and society at large must engage in thoughtful dialogue to navigate these challenges and harness the potential of these innovations responsibly.

Artificial intelligence (AI) is another transformative force reshaping various sectors. From natural language processing and machine learning to computer vision and robotics, AI is enabling machines to perform tasks that once required human intelligence. In healthcare, AI algorithms can analyze medical images with remarkable accuracy, aiding in early diagnosis and treatment planning. In finance, AI-driven trading systems can process vast amounts of data to make informed investment decisions. The potential applications of AI are vast, and its impact on productivity and efficiency is profound.

However, the rise of AI also brings concerns about job displacement and ethical considerations. As machines become capable of performing tasks traditionally done by humans, there is a growing need to reskill and upskill the workforce to adapt to the changing job landscape. Additionally, ensuring that AI systems are transparent, fair, and unbiased is crucial to prevent unintended consequences and discrimination. The development of ethical AI frameworks and guidelines will be essential to address these challenges and build trust in AI technologies.

The intersection of AI and robotics is giving rise to a new generation of intelligent machines. From autonomous drones and robotic assistants to advanced manufacturing robots, these machines are transforming industries and redefining the nature of work. In agriculture, autonomous drones can monitor crop health and optimize irrigation, while robotic harvesters can efficiently pick fruits and vegetables. In manufacturing, collaborative robots, or cobots, work alongside human workers to enhance productivity and precision. The integration of AI and robotics is driving automation to new heights, enabling more efficient and flexible production processes.

In the realm of education, technology is revolutionizing the way we learn and access information. Online learning platforms, virtual classrooms, and AI-powered tutoring systems are making education more accessible and personalized. Students can now learn at their own pace, access a wealth of resources, and receive real-time feedback on their progress. The COVID-19 pandemic has accelerated the adoption of digital learning tools, highlighting the potential of technology to bridge educational gaps and provide lifelong learning opportunities. As educational institutions continue to embrace digital transformation, the future of learning is set to become more inclusive and adaptive.

The entertainment industry is also undergoing a digital revolution. Streaming services, virtual reality experiences, and interactive content are reshaping how we consume media and engage with stories. The rise of streaming platforms has democratized content creation, allowing independent creators to reach global audiences. Virtual reality is offering immersive experiences that transport users to new worlds, while interactive content is enabling viewers to influence the narrative and outcomes of stories. These innovations are not only changing the way we entertain ourselves but also opening new avenues for creative expression and storytelling.

In the world of finance, fintech innovations are disrupting traditional banking and financial services. Digital payment systems, blockchain-based transactions, and AI-driven financial planning tools are making financial services more accessible, efficient, and secure. Mobile banking apps allow users to manage their finances on the go, while blockchain technology is enabling faster and more transparent cross-border transactions. AI-powered robo-advisors are providing personalized investment advice, making wealth management more accessible to a broader audience. The fintech revolution is democratizing finance and empowering individuals to take control of their financial futures.

As we navigate this era of rapid technological change, it is essential to consider the broader societal implications. The digital divide, which refers to the gap between those who have access to digital technologies and those who do not, remains a significant challenge. Ensuring that everyone has access to the benefits of technology, regardless of their socioeconomic status or geographic location, is crucial for fostering inclusive growth and development. Efforts to bridge the digital divide must include investments in infrastructure, digital literacy programs, and policies that promote equitable access to technology.

Moreover, the ethical use of technology is a pressing concern. As we develop and deploy new technologies, we must consider their impact on privacy, security, and human rights. Data privacy is a critical issue, as the proliferation of connected devices and digital services generates vast amounts of personal data. Protecting this data from breaches and misuse is paramount to maintaining trust in technology. Additionally, the ethical implications of technologies such as AI and gene editing must be carefully examined to ensure that they are used responsibly and for the greater good.

The future is undoubtedly exciting, with technological advancements offering unprecedented opportunities for innovation and progress. However, it is also a time of uncertainty and complexity. Navigating this landscape requires a balanced approach that embraces the potential of technology while addressing its challenges and risks. By fostering collaboration, promoting ethical practices, and ensuring equitable access, we can harness the power of technology to create a better, more inclusive future for all.

CHAPTER 10

CODING FOR SPECIALIZED CARE SETTINGS

Outpatient and Ambulatory Coding

Outpatient and ambulatory coding is a specialized area within the medical coding field that focuses on documenting and billing services provided to patients who do not require hospital admission. This type of coding is essential for ensuring that healthcare providers are reimbursed accurately and promptly for their services. It involves translating medical procedures, diagnoses, and treatments into standardized codes used for billing and insurance purposes. The complexity of outpatient and ambulatory coding arises from the need to accurately capture a wide range of services, from routine check-ups to complex diagnostic tests and minor surgical procedures.

The importance of outpatient and ambulatory coding cannot be overstated. Accurate coding ensures that healthcare providers receive appropriate compensation for their services, supporting the financial health of medical practices and facilities. Moreover, precise coding is crucial for maintaining compliance with regulatory requirements and avoiding potential legal issues. Inaccurate or incomplete coding can lead to denied claims, delayed payments, and audits or penalties from insurance companies and government agencies.

One of the critical challenges in outpatient and ambulatory coding is keeping up with the ever-evolving coding systems and guidelines. The primary coding systems used in this field are the International Classification of Diseases, Tenth Revision, Clinical Modification (ICD-10-CM), and the Current Procedural Terminology (CPT) codes. These codes are regularly updated to reflect new medical knowledge, technologies, and procedures. Coders must stay current with these changes to ensure accurate and compliant coding. Additionally, they must be proficient in using coding software and electronic health record (EHR) systems, which are integral to the coding process.

Another critical aspect of outpatient and ambulatory coding is the need for detailed and accurate documentation. Coders rely on the information provided by healthcare providers to assign the correct codes. Incomplete or unclear documentation can lead to coding errors, which can have significant financial and legal implications. Therefore, effective communication and collaboration between coders and healthcare providers are essential. Coders must be able to interpret medical terminology and understand the nuances of various medical procedures and treatments to ensure accurate coding.

The role of outpatient and ambulatory coders extends beyond simply assigning codes. They also play a vital role in ensuring the overall quality and integrity of the medical record. This includes verifying that the documentation supports the codes assigned, identifying discrepancies or inconsistencies, and working with healthcare providers to resolve any issues. Coders must also be vigilant in identifying potential coding errors or fraud and taking appropriate action to address these concerns.

In the ever-changing healthcare landscape, outpatient and ambulatory coders must be adaptable and continuously seek opportunities for professional development. This may involve pursuing additional certifications, attending coding workshops and conferences, and participating in ongoing education and training programs. By staying current with industry trends and best practices, coders can enhance their skills and contribute to the overall efficiency and effectiveness of the healthcare system.

The detailed explanation of outpatient and ambulatory coding delves into this specialized field's specific processes and techniques. Coders must be proficient in using the ICD-10-CM and CPT coding systems, which are the foundation of medical coding. ICD-10-CM codes classify and code diagnoses, symptoms, and other health conditions, while CPT codes describe medical, surgical, and diagnostic procedures and services. These codes are essential for accurately documenting and billing outpatient and ambulatory services.

One of the primary tasks of outpatient and ambulatory coders is to review and analyze medical records to identify the appropriate codes for each service provided. This requires a thorough understanding of medical terminology, anatomy, and physiology and the ability to interpret clinical documentation. Coders must be able to distinguish between similar procedures and diagnoses to assign the most accurate codes. For example, they must differentiate between a routine office visit and a more complex evaluation and management service, each with its codes and billing requirements.

In addition to assigning codes, outpatient and ambulatory coders must ensure that the codes are correctly sequenced and that all relevant codes are included. This is important for accurately reflecting the complexity and scope of the services provided. Coders must also know of any coding guidelines and payer-specific requirements that may impact the coding process. For example, certain insurance companies may have specific rules for coding certain procedures or require additional documentation to support the codes assigned.

Another important aspect of outpatient and ambulatory coding is the use of modifiers. Modifiers are two-digit codes that provide additional information about a procedure or service, such as whether it was performed on a specific body part or a repeat procedure. Modifiers provide more detailed information about services and ensure accurate billing and reimbursement. Coders must be familiar with the various modifiers and their appropriate use to avoid coding errors and potential payment denials.

The outpatient and ambulatory coding review involves a comprehensive analysis of the coding process and its impact on healthcare providers and patients. Accurate coding is essential for ensuring that healthcare providers are reimbursed for their services and that patients receive the care they need. Inaccurate or incomplete coding can lead to significant financial losses for healthcare providers and delays in patient care. It can also result in denied claims, which can be time-consuming and costly to appeal. Therefore, the accuracy and completeness of coding are paramount.

Attention to detail is one of the most critical skills for outpatient and ambulatory coders. Coders must meticulously review medical records and documentation to ensure that all relevant information is captured and accurately coded. This includes verifying that the documentation supports the codes assigned and that any discrepancies or inconsistencies are addressed. Coders must also be vigilant in identifying potential coding errors or fraud and taking appropriate action to address these concerns.

Effective communication and collaboration between coders and healthcare providers are essential for ensuring accurate and compliant coding. Coders must be able to clearly and effectively communicate with healthcare providers to obtain the necessary documentation and clarify any questions or concerns. This may involve working closely with physicians, nurses, and other healthcare professionals to ensure that the documentation accurately reflects the services provided and supports the codes assigned.

In addition to their technical skills, outpatient and ambulatory coders must possess strong analytical and problem-solving abilities. They must be able to analyze complex medical records and documentation to identify the appropriate codes and ensure that all relevant information is captured. This requires a thorough understanding of medical terminology, anatomy, and physiology and the ability to interpret clinical documentation. Coders must also be able to identify and resolve any coding issues or discrepancies, which may involve working with healthcare providers to obtain additional documentation or clarification.

The role of outpatient and ambulatory coders is constantly evolving, and coders must be adaptable and continuously seek opportunities for professional development. This may involve pursuing additional certifications, attending coding workshops and conferences, and participating in ongoing education and training programs. By staying current with industry trends and best practices, coders can enhance their skills and contribute to the overall efficiency and effectiveness of the healthcare system.

Technological advances and changes in healthcare regulations will likely shape the future of outpatient and ambulatory coding. The increasing use of electronic health records (EHRs) and coding software has streamlined the coding process and improved accuracy and efficiency. However, coders must use these technologies proficiently and stay current with updates or changes. Additionally, changes in healthcare regulations and reimbursement policies may impact the coding process, and coders must be aware of these changes and adapt accordingly.

In conclusion, outpatient and ambulatory coding is a specialized and complex field requiring high expertise and attention to detail. Accurate and compliant coding ensures that healthcare providers are reimbursed for their services and that patients receive the care they need. Coders must possess strong technical skills, analytical abilities, and effective communication and collaboration skills to succeed in this field. By staying current with industry trends and best practices, coders can contribute to the overall efficiency and effectiveness of the healthcare system and ensure the financial health of medical practices and facilities.

Inpatient Hospital Facility Coding

Inpatient hospital facility coding is a specialized area within the medical coding profession that requires a deep understanding of various coding systems, medical terminology, and healthcare regulations. This type of coding involves assigning codes to diagnoses, procedures, and services provided to patients during their stay in a hospital. The accuracy and completeness of these codes are crucial for proper reimbursement, compliance with regulations, and the overall quality of patient care.

Inpatient coding is distinct from outpatient coding in several ways. While outpatient coding typically involves coding for services provided in a single visit, inpatient coding encompasses a patient's hospital stay. This means that inpatient coders must review and code a comprehensive set of medical records, including admission notes, progress notes, operative reports, discharge summaries, and more. The complexity of inpatient coding requires coders to thoroughly understand the International Classification of Diseases, Tenth Revision, Clinical Modification (ICD-10-CM) and the International Classification of Diseases, Tenth Revision, Procedure Coding System (ICD-10-PCS).

One of the primary challenges in inpatient coding is ensuring that all relevant diagnoses and procedures are accurately captured and coded. This requires coders to meticulously review the medical records and documentation to identify all conditions present on admission and any complications or comorbidities that developed during the hospital stay. Coders must also be able to distinguish between principal diagnoses, which are the main reasons for the patient's admission, and secondary diagnoses, which are additional conditions that affect patient care.

In addition to coding for diagnoses, inpatient coders must assign codes for procedures performed during the hospital stay. This includes surgical procedures, diagnostic tests, and therapeutic interventions. The ICD-10-PCS coding system is used for this purpose, and it requires coders to have a detailed understanding of the anatomy, physiology, and specific techniques used in various medical procedures. Coders must also be familiar with the guidelines and conventions of the ICD-10-PCS system to ensure accurate and consistent coding.

The role of inpatient coders is not limited to assigning codes. They also play a critical role in ensuring healthcare regulations and guidelines compliance. This includes adhering to the coding guidelines established by the Centers for Medicare & Medicaid Services (CMS) and other regulatory bodies. Coders must also be vigilant in identifying potential coding errors, fraud, or abuse and taking appropriate action to address these issues. This may involve working closely with healthcare providers, auditors, and compliance officers to ensure the coding practices are accurate and compliant.

Effective communication and collaboration are essential for inpatient coders. They must clearly and effectively communicate with healthcare providers to obtain the necessary documentation and clarify any questions or concerns. This may involve working closely with physicians, nurses, and other healthcare professionals to ensure that the documentation accurately reflects the services provided and supports the codes assigned. Coders must also be able to explain coding guidelines and regulations to healthcare providers and assist them in understanding the importance of accurate and complete documentation.

Inpatient coders must possess strong analytical and problem-solving skills. They must be able to analyze complex medical records and documentation to identify the appropriate codes and ensure that all relevant information is captured. This requires a thorough understanding of medical terminology, anatomy, and physiology and the ability to interpret clinical documentation. Coders must also be able to identify and resolve any coding issues or discrepancies, which may involve working with healthcare providers to obtain additional documentation or clarification.

The role of inpatient coders is constantly evolving, and coders must be adaptable and continuously seek opportunities for professional development. This may involve pursuing additional certifications, attending coding workshops and conferences, and participating in ongoing education and training programs. By staying current with industry trends and best practices, coders can enhance their skills and contribute to the overall efficiency and effectiveness of the healthcare system.

The future of inpatient coding is likely to be shaped by advances in technology and changes in healthcare regulations. The increasing use of electronic health records (EHRs) and coding software has streamlined the coding process and improved accuracy and efficiency. However, coders must use these technologies proficiently and stay current with updates or changes. Additionally, changes in healthcare regulations and reimbursement policies may impact the coding process, and coders must be aware of these changes and adapt accordingly.

Inpatient hospital facility coding is a specialized and complex field requiring high expertise and attention to detail. Accurate and compliant coding ensures that healthcare providers are reimbursed for their services and that patients receive the care they need. Coders must possess strong technical skills, analytical abilities, and effective communication and collaboration skills to succeed in this field. By staying current with industry trends and best practices, coders can contribute to the overall efficiency and effectiveness of the healthcare system and ensure the financial health of medical practices and facilities.

The importance of inpatient coding cannot be overstated. It serves as the backbone of hospital billing and reimbursement processes. Hospitals need accurate coding to avoid significant financial losses, which can impact their ability to provide quality care. Moreover, precise coding is essential for maintaining compliance with healthcare regulations and avoiding potential legal repercussions. Coders must navigate a labyrinth of guidelines, rules, and regulations, ensuring that every code assigned aligns with the clinical documentation and meets the stringent requirements set forth by regulatory bodies.

The financial implications of inpatient coding extend beyond reimbursement. Accurate coding is also pivotal in hospital performance metrics, quality reporting, and public health data. Hospitals rely on coded data to track patient outcomes, identify trends, and implement quality improvement initiatives. Public health agencies also use this data to monitor disease prevalence, assess the effectiveness of interventions, and allocate resources. Inaccurate coding can skew these metrics, leading to misguided policies and resource allocation.

Inpatient coders must also be adept at navigating the nuances of coding for different payer systems. Medicare, Medicaid, and private insurers each have their own rules and requirements for coding and billing. Coders must be familiar with these variations and ensure that the codes assigned meet the specific criteria for each payer. This requires a deep understanding of payer policies and staying current with changes or updates.

The transition to value-based care has further emphasized the importance of accurate inpatient coding. Under value-based care models, reimbursement is tied to the quality and efficiency of care rather than the service volume. Correct coding is essential for capturing the complexity of patient care and ensuring that hospitals are fairly compensated for their services. Coders must be able to identify and code for all relevant conditions and procedures, including those that impact patient outcomes and resource utilization.

Inpatient coders are critical in supporting clinical documentation improvement (CDI) initiatives. CDI programs aim to enhance the accuracy and completeness of clinical documentation, ensuring that it accurately reflects the patient's clinical status and the care provided. Coders work closely with CDI specialists to identify documentation gaps, provide feedback to healthcare providers, and ensure that the documentation supports the assigned codes. This collaboration is essential for improving the quality of clinical documentation and ensuring accurate coding and reimbursement.

The complexity of inpatient coding requires coders to possess a unique blend of technical skills, clinical knowledge, and critical thinking abilities. They must be able to interpret complex medical records, identify relevant diagnoses and procedures, and apply the appropriate codes. This requires a deep understanding of medical terminology, anatomy, and physiology and staying current with coding guidelines and updates. Coders must also be able to think critically and problem-solvers, identifying and resolving any coding issues or discrepancies.

Inpatient coders must also be detail-oriented and meticulous in their work. Coding accuracy depends on the coder's ability to precisely review and analyze medical records, ensuring that all relevant information is captured and coded correctly. Even minor errors in coding can have significant financial and compliance implications, making attention to detail a critical skill for inpatient coders.

The role of inpatient coders is dynamic; it constantly evolves in response to changes in healthcare delivery, technology, and regulations. Coders must be adaptable and committed to continuous learning and professional development. This may involve pursuing additional certifications, attending coding workshops and conferences, and participating in ongoing education and training programs. By staying current with industry trends and best practices, coders can enhance their skills and contribute to the overall efficiency and effectiveness of the healthcare system.

Inpatient hospital facility coding is a vital and complex field requiring high expertise and attention to detail. Accurate and compliant coding is essential for ensuring that healthcare providers are reimbursed for their services, maintaining compliance with regulations, and supporting quality improvement initiatives. Coders must possess strong technical skills, clinical knowledge, and critical thinking abilities to succeed. By staying current with industry trends and best practices, coders can contribute to the overall efficiency and effectiveness of the healthcare system and ensure the financial health of medical practices and facilities.

Physician Practice and Clinic Coding

Physician practice and clinic coding are critical to the healthcare system, ensuring that medical services are accurately documented and appropriately reimbursed. This process involves translating clinical documentation into standardized codes that reflect the diagnoses, procedures, and services provided during patient encounters. These codes are used by insurance companies to determine reimbursement rates, by healthcare providers to track patient care, and by public health agencies to monitor disease trends and outcomes.

The importance of accurate coding cannot be overstated. It directly impacts the financial health of medical practices and clinics, influencing their ability to receive timely and appropriate payments for their services. Inaccurate coding can lead to claim denials, delayed payments, and potential audits, all of which can strain the resources of a practice. Moreover, coding errors can affect patient care by misrepresenting the clinical picture, leading to inappropriate treatment decisions or gaps in care continuity.

Physician practice and clinic coding are governed by complex rules and guidelines, including the International Classification of Diseases (ICD) codes for diagnoses, and the Current Procedural Terminology (CPT) codes for procedures and services. Coders must be well-versed in these coding systems and the specific requirements of different payers, such as Medicare, Medicaid, and private insurers. This requires ongoing education and training to stay current with updates and changes in coding guidelines.

The role of a coder in a physician practice or clinic extends beyond simply assigning codes. Coders must also ensure that the clinical documentation supports the codes assigned and clearly and accurately represents the patient's condition and the care provided. This often involves working closely with healthcare providers to clarify documentation, address discrepancies, and capture all relevant information. Effective communication and collaboration between coders and providers are essential for accurate coding and optimal patient care.

In addition to coding for reimbursement, physician practice and clinic coders play a vital role in quality reporting and performance measurement. Many healthcare organizations participate in quality improvement programs requiring coded data submission to track performance metrics, such as patient outcomes, adherence to clinical guidelines, and patient satisfaction. Accurate coding is essential for these programs, ensuring the submitted data reflects the quality of care and supports efforts to improve patient outcomes.

The transition to value-based care has further emphasized the importance of accurate coding in physician practices and clinics. Under value-based care models, reimbursement is tied to the quality and efficiency of care rather than the service volume. This requires coders to capture the full complexity of patient care, including all relevant diagnoses and procedures, to ensure that providers are fairly compensated for the care they deliver. Coders must also be able to identify and code for social determinants of health, which can impact patient outcomes and resource utilization.

Physician practice and clinic coders must possess a unique blend of technical skills, clinical knowledge, and critical thinking abilities. They must be able to interpret complex medical records, identify relevant diagnoses and procedures, and apply the appropriate codes. This requires a deep understanding of medical terminology, anatomy, and physiology and staying current with coding guidelines and updates. Coders must also be able to think critically and problem-solvers, identifying and resolving any coding issues or discrepancies.

The complexity of physician practice and clinic coding requires coders to be detail-oriented and meticulous. Coding accuracy depends on the coder's ability to precisely review and analyze medical records, ensuring that all relevant information is captured and coded correctly. Even minor errors in coding can have significant financial and compliance implications, making attention to detail a critical skill for coders.

The role of physician practice and clinic coders is not static; it is constantly evolving in response to changes in healthcare delivery, technology, and regulations. Coders must be adaptable and committed to continuous learning and professional development. This may involve pursuing additional certifications, attending coding workshops and conferences, and participating in ongoing education and training programs. By staying current with industry trends and best practices, coders can enhance their skills and contribute to the overall efficiency and effectiveness of the healthcare system.

Physician practice and clinic coding is a vital and complex field requiring high expertise and attention to detail. Accurate and compliant coding is essential for ensuring that healthcare providers are reimbursed for their services, maintaining compliance with regulations, and supporting quality improvement initiatives. Coders must possess strong technical skills, clinical knowledge, and critical thinking abilities to succeed. By staying current with industry trends and best practices, coders can contribute to the overall efficiency and effectiveness of the healthcare system and ensure the financial health of medical practices and clinics.

The financial implications of physician practice and clinic coding extend beyond reimbursement. Accurate coding is also pivotal in practice performance metrics, quality reporting, and public health data. Practices rely on coded data to track patient outcomes, identify trends, and implement quality improvement initiatives. Public health agencies also use this data to monitor disease prevalence, assess the effectiveness of interventions, and allocate resources. Inaccurate coding can skew these metrics, leading to misguided policies and resource allocation.

Risk Adjustment and Hierarchical Condition Categories

Risk adjustment and hierarchical condition categories (HCCs) are pivotal concepts in healthcare finance and management. These mechanisms ensure that healthcare providers adequately compensate for the patients' complexity and severity. By understanding these concepts, healthcare professionals can better navigate the financial landscape, ensuring that resources are allocated efficiently and equitably.

Risk adjustment is a statistical process that adjusts payments and performance metrics to account for patients' health status and related costs. This process is essential in environments where providers are paid based on the health outcomes of their patients, such as in value-based care models. Without risk adjustment, providers who treat sicker, more complex patients would be unfairly penalized, as their patients are inherently more likely to have worse outcomes and higher costs. By incorporating risk adjustment, these models can more accurately reflect the true performance of healthcare providers, ensuring that those who take on more challenging cases are not disadvantaged.

Hierarchical condition categories (HCCs) are a specific risk adjustment method used primarily in the Medicare Advantage program. HCCs categorize patients based on their diagnoses, with each category assigned a particular weight that reflects the expected cost of care for patients within that category. These weights are then used to adjust payments to healthcare providers, ensuring that those who treat patients with more severe or complex conditions receive higher compensation. The HCC model is hierarchical because it groups related conditions together, with more severe conditions subsuming less severe ones. For example, a patient with both diabetes and a more severe condition like end-stage renal disease would be categorized based on the more severe condition, as it encompasses the costs and complexities of managing the less severe one.

The implementation of HCCs involves several steps. First, patient diagnoses are collected from medical records and claims data. These diagnoses are then mapped to specific HCCs using a predefined algorithm. Each HCC is assigned a weight based on historical cost data, which reflects the average cost of treating patients within that category. These weights are then summed to produce a risk score for each patient, which is used to adjust payments to healthcare providers. This process ensures that providers are compensated fairly for the complexity and severity of their patients, promoting equity and efficiency in the healthcare system.

The importance of accurate and comprehensive documentation cannot be overstated in the context of HCCs. Providers must ensure that all relevant diagnoses are captured and documented in the medical record, as missing or incomplete information can lead to inaccurate risk scores and, consequently, inadequate compensation. This requires a collaborative effort between clinicians, coders, and administrative staff to ensure that documentation practices are robust and consistent. Regular training and education on the importance of accurate documentation and coding can help mitigate these challenges, ensuring that providers receive appropriate compensation for their care.

In addition to ensuring fair compensation, risk adjustment and HCCs also play a crucial role in quality measurement and performance evaluation. By adjusting for patients' health status and related costs, these mechanisms allow for more accurate comparisons of provider performance. This is particularly important in value-based care models, where providers are incentivized to improve the quality and efficiency of care. Without risk adjustment, providers who treat sicker, more complex patients would be unfairly penalized, as their patients are inherently more likely to have worse outcomes and higher costs. By incorporating risk adjustment, these models can more accurately reflect the true performance of healthcare providers, ensuring that those who take on more challenging cases are not disadvantaged.

The use of HCCs in the Medicare Advantage program has been associated with several benefits. By ensuring that payments are adjusted based on the complexity and severity of patients' conditions, HCCs promote equity and efficiency in the healthcare system. Providers who treat more complex patients receive higher compensation, which helps to offset the additional costs and resources required to manage these patients.

This, in turn, can help reduce disparities in access to care, as providers are more willing to take on challenging cases when adequately compensated for their efforts.

However, the implementation of HCCs is not without challenges. One of the primary concerns is the potential for gaming or manipulating the system. Providers may be incentivized to upcode or exaggerate the severity of patients' conditions to receive higher payments. To mitigate this risk, robust auditing and oversight mechanisms are essential. Regular audits of medical records and claims data can help to identify and address instances of upcoding or other forms of fraud, ensuring that the system remains fair and accurate.

Another challenge is the complexity of the HCC model itself. With numerous categories and weights to consider, mapping diagnoses to HCCs can be time-consuming and prone to errors. This requires high expertise and attention to detail from coders and administrative staff. Investing in training and education on the HCC model can help to ensure that staff are well-equipped to navigate this complexity, reducing the risk of errors and inaccuracies.

Despite these challenges, the benefits of risk adjustment and HCCs are clear. By ensuring that payments are adjusted based on the complexity and severity of patients' conditions, these mechanisms promote equity and efficiency within the healthcare system. Providers are more likely to accept and adequately treat patients with complex conditions when they know their efforts will be fairly compensated. This can improve patient outcomes, as those with severe or multiple conditions receive the necessary comprehensive care.

Moreover, risk adjustment and HCCs facilitate more accurate benchmarking and performance comparisons among healthcare providers. By accounting for the varying levels of patient complexity, these mechanisms allow for a more level playing field. Providers can be evaluated based on the quality of care they deliver rather than the inherent risk profiles of their patient populations. This fosters a culture of continuous improvement as providers strive to enhance care quality and efficiency without being penalized for taking on more challenging cases.

Integrating advanced data analytics and machine learning into the risk adjustment process holds promise for further refining these mechanisms. By leveraging large datasets and sophisticated algorithms, healthcare organizations can develop more precise models that better capture the nuances of patient complexity and associated costs. This can lead to more accurate risk scores and more equitable payment adjustments. Additionally, predictive analytics can help identify patients at high risk of adverse outcomes, enabling proactive interventions to improve care quality and reduce costs.

Collaboration and communication among stakeholders are crucial for successfully implementing risk adjustment and HCCs. Healthcare providers, payers, policymakers, and technology vendors must work together to develop and refine these mechanisms. Open dialogue and shared learning can help address challenges, identify best practices, and drive continuous improvement. For instance, regular feedback loops between providers and payers can help identify areas where documentation practices can be enhanced, ensuring that risk scores accurately reflect patient complexity.

The role of technology in supporting risk adjustment and HCCs cannot be overstated. Electronic health records (EHRs) and health information exchanges (HIEs) are critical in capturing and sharing patient data. Advanced coding and documentation tools can streamline the process of mapping diagnoses to HCCs, reducing the risk of errors and improving efficiency. Additionally, decision support systems can provide real-time guidance to clinicians, helping them ensure that all relevant diagnoses are captured and documented accurately.

Education and training are essential to a successful risk adjustment and HCC strategy. Clinicians, coders, and administrative staff must understand inaccurate documentation, coding principles, and practices. Regular training sessions, workshops, and continuing education programs can help ensure that staff are up-to-date with the latest guidelines and best practices. This improves the accuracy of risk scores and enhances the overall quality of patient care.

The ethical considerations surrounding risk adjustment and HCCs are also worth noting. While these mechanisms promote fairness and equity, they must be implemented to avoid unintended consequences. For instance, providers may focus disproportionately on coding and documentation at the expense of patient care. It is essential to balance accurate documentation and to deliver high-quality, patient-centred care to mitigate this. Ethical guidelines and oversight mechanisms can ensure that the focus remains on improving patient outcomes while maintaining the integrity of the risk adjustment process.

In conclusion, risk adjustment and hierarchical condition categories are vital tools in modern healthcare. These mechanisms promote equity, efficiency, and quality in healthcare delivery by ensuring that payments and performance metrics accurately reflect the complexity and severity of patients' conditions. While challenges exist, ongoing collaboration, education, and technological innovation can help address these issues and enhance the effectiveness of risk adjustment and HCCs. As the healthcare industry evolves, these mechanisms will play an increasingly important role in ensuring that providers are fairly compensated for their care, ultimately leading to better patient outcomes and a more sustainable healthcare system.

CHAPTER 11

ADVANCED CODING CONCEPTS AND CASE STUDIES

Coding Complexities and Challenges

Navigating the intricate world of coding complexities and challenges can feel like traversing a labyrinth. The landscape is ever-evolving, with new languages, frameworks, and paradigms emerging rapidly. For beginners, this can be both exciting and overwhelming. The allure of creating something from nothing, of solving problems with elegant lines of code, is a powerful motivator. Yet, the path is fraught with obstacles that can derail even the most determined novice. Understanding these complexities and challenges is crucial for anyone embarking on a coding journey.

One of the primary complexities in coding is the sheer variety of programming languages available. Each language has its own syntax, semantics, and use cases. For instance, Python is renowned for its simplicity and readability, making it a popular choice for beginners. On the other hand, languages like C++ offer more control over system resources but come with a steeper learning curve. Choosing the correct language for a specific task requires a deep understanding of the problem at hand and the strengths and weaknesses of each language.

Another significant challenge is debugging. Writing code is only half the battle; ensuring it works as intended is an entirely different beast. Bugs can be elusive, often hiding in the most unexpected places. They can stem from simple typographical errors or more complex logical flaws. Effective debugging requires a systematic approach, patience, and a keen eye for detail. Tools like debuggers and integrated development environments (IDEs) can aid in this process, but the coder's intuition and experience play a pivotal role.

The complexity of algorithms and data structures also poses a considerable challenge. These are the building blocks of efficient and effective code. Understanding how to implement and optimize algorithms and how to choose the proper data structure for a given problem is essential. This requires not only theoretical knowledge but also practical experience. Beginners often struggle with these concepts, but mastering them is crucial for tackling more advanced coding tasks.

Collaboration and version control adds another layer of complexity. In a professional setting, coding is rarely a solitary activity. Developers must work together, often on the same codebase, which necessitates clear communication and coordination. Version control systems like Git are indispensable tools in this regard. They allow multiple developers to work on the same project simultaneously, track changes, and revert to previous versions if needed. However, for beginners, mastering these tools and the associated workflows can take time.

The rapid pace of technological advancement means that coders must be lifelong learners. New languages, frameworks, and tools are constantly being developed, and staying current is a perpetual challenge. This requires a commitment to continuous learning and professional development. Online courses, coding boot camps, and developer communities can provide valuable resources and support, but the bonus is on the individual to stay informed and adapt to new developments.

Understanding the intricacies of coding complexities and challenges is only the beginning. Delving deeper, one must grapple with the nuances of different programming paradigms. Procedural programming, object-oriented programming, functional programming—each paradigm offers a unique approach to problem-solving.

Procedural programming, for instance, focuses on a sequence of instructions to perform a task, while object-oriented programming organizes code into objects that represent real-world entities. On the other hand, functional programming emphasizes using pure functions and immutable data. Each paradigm has its principles and best practices, and choosing the right one for a given problem requires a nuanced understanding of its strengths and weaknesses.

Error handling is another critical aspect of coding that presents its own set of challenges. Errors are inevitable, but how they are handled can make the difference between a robust, user-friendly application and a frustrating, unreliable one. Effective error handling involves anticipating potential issues, providing meaningful error messages, and ensuring the application can recover gracefully. This requires a proactive approach and a thorough understanding of the possible pitfalls in the code.

Security is a paramount concern in coding, particularly in today's interconnected world. Writing secure code involves more than just following best practices; it requires a deep understanding of potential vulnerabilities and how to mitigate them. This includes protecting against common threats like SQL injection, cross-site scripting (XSS), and buffer overflows. Security must be considered at every stage of the development process, from design to deployment, and requires ongoing vigilance to stay ahead of emerging threats.

Performance optimization is another area where coding complexities come to the fore. Writing code that works is one thing; writing code that works efficiently is another. Performance optimization involves identifying bottlenecks, understanding the underlying hardware and software architecture, and making informed trade-offs between speed, memory usage, and other resources. This requires analytical skills, practical experience, and a deep understanding of the application's requirements.

The human element must be considered when discussing coding complexities and challenges. Coding is as much an art as a science, and the coder's mindset, creativity, and problem-solving skills play a crucial role. Overcoming coding challenges often requires thinking outside the box, experimenting with different approaches, and learning from failures. The ability to persevere in the face of setbacks, remain curious, seek out new knowledge, and adapt to changing circumstances are all essential traits for a successful coder. The journey is as much about personal growth and development as it is about technical proficiency.

Documentation is another often overlooked aspect of coding that can present significant challenges. Writing clear, concise, and comprehensive documentation is crucial for maintaining and scaling a codebase. Good documentation is a roadmap for other developers, helping them understand the code's structure, functionality, and intended use. It also aids in debugging and future development. However, writing adequate documentation requires a balance between technical detail and readability, and it often demands as much skill and effort as writing the code itself.

The user experience (UX) is a critical consideration in coding, particularly for applications that interact directly with end-users. Creating a seamless, intuitive, and enjoyable user experience requires a deep understanding of human-computer interaction principles and empathy for the user's needs and preferences. This involves designing an aesthetically pleasing interface and ensuring the application is responsive, accessible, and easy to navigate. Achieving this balance can be challenging, mainly when dealing with complex functionality or diverse user groups.

Testing is another crucial aspect of coding that presents its own set of challenges. Writing tests to ensure the code behaves as expected under various conditions is essential for maintaining code quality and reliability. This includes unit tests, which test individual code components, and integration tests, which ensure that different elements work together correctly. Writing practical tests requires a thorough understanding of the code's functionality and potential edge cases and a commitment to maintaining and updating the tests as the code evolves.

The ethical implications of coding cannot be ignored. Coders are responsible for considering their work's broader impact on society. This includes issues related to privacy, security, and fairness. For example, algorithms used in decision-making processes must be designed to avoid bias and ensure transparency. Similarly, applications that handle sensitive data must prioritize user privacy and security. Navigating these ethical considerations requires technical expertise, moral awareness, and a commitment to responsible coding practices.

The role of mentorship and community support in overcoming coding challenges cannot be overstated. Learning to code can be a daunting and isolating experience, but having access to experienced mentors and supportive communities can make a significant difference. Mentors can provide guidance, share their experiences, and offer valuable feedback, while communities can offer a sense of camaraderie and shared purpose. Engaging with these resources can help beginners navigate the complexities of coding and build the confidence and skills needed to succeed.

The journey of mastering coding complexities and challenges is a continuous one. It requires a commitment to lifelong learning, a willingness to embrace new technologies and methodologies, and a dedication to honing one's skills. The rewards, however, are well worth the effort. Coding offers the opportunity to create, innovate, and solve problems that can profoundly impact the world. The journey can be incredibly fulfilling and rewarding for those willing to embrace the challenges and complexities.

Coding Audits and Compliance Reviews

Coding audits and compliance reviews are essential to maintaining software systems' integrity and reliability. These processes ensure the code adheres to established standards, regulations, and best practices, minimizing risks and enhancing overall quality. Understanding the importance and methodology of coding audits and compliance reviews can be daunting for beginners, yet it is crucial for developing robust and secure applications.

Coding audits involve thoroughly examining the codebase to identify potential issues, such as security vulnerabilities, performance bottlenecks, and adherence to coding standards. This process often includes both automated tools and manual inspections. Automated tools can quickly scan large codebases for common issues, while manual inspections allow for a more nuanced understanding of the code's structure and logic. The goal is to ensure that the code is functional but also maintainable, scalable, and secure.

Compliance reviews, on the other hand, focus on ensuring that the code meets specific regulatory requirements and industry standards. These reviews are critical in healthcare, finance, and telecommunications industries, where non-compliance can result in severe penalties and reputational damage. Compliance reviews often involve checking for adherence to data protection regulations, such as GDPR or HIPAA, and industry-specific standards like PCI-DSS for payment processing.

Conducting coding audits and compliance reviews can be broken down into several key steps. First, it is essential to establish a clear set of criteria and standards against which the code will be evaluated. This may include internal coding guidelines, industry best practices, and relevant regulatory requirements. Next, the codebase is analyzed using automated tools and manual inspections. Automated tools can quickly identify common issues like code smells, security vulnerabilities, and performance bottlenecks. On the other hand, manual inspections allow for a more in-depth understanding of the code's structure and logic, enabling the identification of more subtle issues.

Once the analysis is complete, the findings are documented and prioritized based on their severity and potential impact. This documentation serves as a roadmap for addressing the identified issues and improving the overall quality of the code.

To ensure the findings are understood and addressed appropriately, involving all relevant stakeholders in this process, including developers, project managers, and compliance officers, is essential.

Addressing the identified issues often involves a combination of refactoring, optimization, and remediation. Refactoring aims to improve the code's structure and readability without altering its functionality, making it easier to maintain and extend. Optimization focuses on enhancing the code's performance, ensuring it runs efficiently and effectively. Remediation, however, involves fixing security vulnerabilities and other critical issues that could pose a risk to the application and its users.

Regular coding audits and compliance reviews are essential for maintaining the integrity and reliability of software systems. Organizations can minimize risks, enhance code quality, and ensure compliance with relevant regulations and standards by identifying and addressing potential issues early in development. This proactive approach improves the code's overall quality and helps build trust with users and stakeholders, demonstrating a commitment to security, reliability, and best practices.

The benefits of coding audits and compliance reviews extend beyond simply identifying and addressing issues. These processes also provide valuable insights into development, highlighting improvement areas and optimization opportunities. For example, a coding audit may reveal that certain coding practices are leading to performance bottlenecks or security vulnerabilities, prompting a review and revision of internal coding guidelines. Similarly, a compliance review may uncover gaps in the organization's understanding of regulatory requirements, leading to additional training and education for developers and other stakeholders.

In addition to improving code quality and compliance, regular audits and reviews can enhance collaboration and communication within the development team and improve code quality and compliance. By involving all relevant stakeholders in the process, organizations can foster a culture of continuous improvement and shared responsibility for code quality and compliance. This collaborative approach helps ensure that issues are addressed promptly and effectively and promotes a sense of ownership and accountability among team members.

Understanding the importance and methodology of coding audits and compliance reviews can be challenging for beginners, but it is crucial to developing robust and secure applications. By familiarizing themselves with these processes' essential steps and best practices, beginners can develop the skills and knowledge to contribute to high-quality, compliant codebases. This includes learning how to use automated tools for code analysis, understanding the principles of manual code inspections, and staying up-to-date with relevant regulations and industry standards.

One practical approach for beginners is conducting small-scale audits and reviews on their code or open-source projects. This hands-on experience can help to build confidence and competence in identifying and addressing potential issues. Additionally, seeking mentorship and guidance from more experienced developers can provide valuable insights and feedback, helping beginners refine their skills and understanding.

Another important aspect for beginners is to stay informed about the latest developments in coding standards, best practices, and regulatory requirements. This can be achieved through continuous learning and professional development, such as attending workshops, conferences, and online courses. By staying up-to-date with the latest trends and advancements, beginners can ensure that their skills and knowledge remain relevant and effective in maintaining high-quality codebases.

Engaging with the broader developer community can also be beneficial. Participating in forums, discussion groups, and online communities allows beginners to share experiences, ask questions, and learn from others' successes and challenges. This collaborative environment fosters continuous learning and improvement, essential for staying current with best practices and emerging trends.

Another critical aspect is understanding the tools and techniques used in coding audits and compliance reviews. Familiarity with static code analysis tools, such as SonarQube, ESLint, and Checkmarx, can significantly streamline the audit process by automating the detection of everyday issues. These tools can identify code smells, security vulnerabilities, and performance bottlenecks, providing actionable insights that can be addressed during development. Learning to conduct manual code reviews effectively is crucial for identifying more subtle issues that automated tools may miss. This involves understanding code readability, maintainability, and adherence to coding standards.

For compliance reviews, it is essential to have a thorough understanding of the relevant regulations and industry standards that apply to the specific domain. This may include data protection regulations like GDPR or HIPAA, industry-specific standards such as PCI-DSS for payment processing, and internal policies and guidelines. Staying informed about changes and updates to these regulations is crucial for ensuring ongoing compliance and avoiding potential penalties.

Incorporating coding audits and compliance reviews into the development workflow can also enhance the overall efficiency and effectiveness of the process. By integrating these practices into the continuous integration and continuous deployment (CI/CD) pipeline, organizations can ensure that code is regularly reviewed and validated against established standards and regulations. This proactive approach helps identify and address issues early in development, reducing the risk of costly and time-consuming rework.

Moreover, fostering a culture of quality and compliance within the development team is essential for the long-term success of coding audits and compliance reviews. This involves promoting the importance of these practices, providing training and resources to support their implementation, and recognizing and rewarding efforts to improve code quality and compliance. Organizations can ensure that these practices become an integral part of the development process by creating an environment where quality and compliance are prioritized.

For beginners, it is essential to approach coding audits and compliance reviews with a mindset of continuous improvement and learning. Embracing feedback, seeking growth opportunities, and learning new tools and techniques can help build the skills and knowledge needed to contribute effectively to high-quality, compliant codebases. Additionally, developing strong communication and collaboration skills can enhance the ability to work effectively with other team members and stakeholders, ensuring that issues are addressed promptly and effectively.

Coding audits and compliance reviews are essential to maintaining software systems' integrity and reliability. By understanding the importance and methodology of these processes, beginners can develop the skills and knowledge needed to contribute to robust and secure applications. This involves learning how to use automated tools for code analysis, conducting effective manual code reviews, staying informed about relevant regulations and industry standards, and fostering a culture of quality and compliance within the development team. Through continuous learning and collaboration, beginners can play a crucial role in ensuring the ongoing success of coding audits and compliance reviews.

Reimbursement Methodologies

Reimbursement methodologies are crucial in the healthcare industry, determining how providers are compensated for their services. Understanding these methodologies is essential for healthcare management, finance, or policy-making. The reimbursement landscape is complex, influenced by various factors such as regulatory changes, technological advancements, and evolving patient needs. For beginners, grasping the fundamentals of reimbursement methodologies can be challenging but is vital for ensuring financial sustainability and delivering quality care.

Healthcare reimbursement methodologies have evolved significantly over the years. Initially, providers were paid on a fee-for-service basis, where each service rendered was billed separately. This model, while straightforward, often led to inefficiencies and higher costs, as there was little incentive to control spending or improve patient outcomes. Over time, alternative reimbursement models emerged to address these issues and promote value-based care.

One of the most significant shifts in reimbursement methodologies has been the move towards value-based care. This approach rewards providers for care quality and efficiency rather than the service volume. Value-based reimbursement models include pay-for-performance, bundled payments, and accountable care organizations (ACOs). Each model has criteria and metrics for evaluating provider performance and determining compensation.

Pay-for-performance models incentivize providers to meet specific quality and efficiency benchmarks. These benchmarks may include patient satisfaction scores, adherence to clinical guidelines, and reductions in hospital readmissions. Providers who meet or exceed these benchmarks receive financial bonuses, while those who fall short may face penalties. This model encourages continuous improvement and accountability, leading to better patient outcomes.

Bundled payments, also known as episode-based payments, involve a single, comprehensive payment for all services related to a specific episode of care. For example, a bundled payment for a knee replacement surgery would cover pre-operative consultations, the surgery itself, post-operative care, and rehabilitation. This model encourages providers to coordinate care and manage resources efficiently, as they are financially responsible for any cost overruns. By aligning incentives across the care continuum, bundled payments can reduce unnecessary spending and improve patient outcomes.

Accountable care organizations (ACOs) are providers who voluntarily come together to deliver coordinated, high-quality care to a specific patient population. ACOs are rewarded for achieving cost savings and meeting quality benchmarks, with shared savings distributed among the participating providers. This model fosters collaboration and emphasizes preventive care, reducing the need for costly interventions and hospitalizations.

Understanding these reimbursement methodologies requires a comprehensive review of their underlying principles and practical implications. Fee-for-service remains prevalent in many settings, particularly for outpatient and speciality care. However, its limitations are increasingly recognized, prompting a shift towards value-based models. Fee-for-service can lead to fragmented care, as providers are incentivized to maximize the volume of services rather than focusing on patient outcomes. This model also contributes to rising healthcare costs, as there is little emphasis on cost containment or efficiency.

In contrast, value-based reimbursement models prioritize patient outcomes and cost-effectiveness. Pay-for-performance models, for instance, tie financial incentives to specific quality metrics, encouraging providers to deliver high-quality care. These metrics may include patient satisfaction scores, adherence to clinical guidelines, and reductions in hospital readmissions. By linking compensation to performance, pay-for-performance models promote accountability and continuous improvement.

The transition to value-based reimbursement methodologies is not without challenges. Providers must invest in infrastructure, such as electronic health records (EHRs) and data analytics, to track performance metrics and coordinate care. Additionally, there may be resistance to change, as providers accustomed to fee-for-service models hesitate to adopt new approaches. Education and training are essential to help providers understand the benefits of value-based care and how to implement these models effectively.

Moreover, regulatory and policy changes can impact reimbursement methodologies. For example, the Centers for Medicare & Medicaid Services (CMS) has introduced several initiatives to promote value-based care, such as the Medicare Shared Savings Program (MSSP) for ACOs and the Comprehensive Care for Joint Replacement (CJR) model for bundled payments. Staying informed about these changes and adapting to new requirements is crucial for providers to remain compliant and maximize their reimbursement potential.

In conclusion, reimbursement methodologies are critical to healthcare finance, influencing how providers are compensated and care delivered. The shift from fee-for-service to value-based models reflects a broader emphasis on quality, efficiency, and patient outcomes. This transition is driven by the need to control rising healthcare costs while ensuring patients receive the best care. Understanding and adapting to these reimbursement methodologies will be essential for healthcare providers, administrators, and policymakers as the industry evolves.

Data Analysis and Reporting

Data analysis and reporting are crucial in modern decision-making and strategic planning. The ability to interpret and present data effectively can significantly impact the success of an organization. Data analysis involves examining raw data to draw meaningful insights while reporting and communicating these insights clearly and promptly. Together, they form the backbone of informed decision-making, enabling organizations to identify trends, measure performance, and make data-driven decisions.

In today's data-driven world, the sheer volume of data generated daily is staggering. Data is everywhere, from customer transactions and social media interactions to sensor readings and financial records. However, raw data is not valuable until it is analyzed and transformed into actionable insights. This is where data analysis comes into play. Analysts can uncover patterns, correlations, and anomalies within the data by applying various statistical, mathematical, and computational techniques. These insights can inform business strategies, optimize operations, and drive innovation.

Practical data analysis requires a combination of technical skills and domain knowledge. Analysts must be proficient in using tools and software for data manipulation, visualization, and statistical analysis. They must also deeply understand the specific industry or domain they are working in, as this context is essential for interpreting the data accurately. For example, a healthcare analyst must understand medical terminology and healthcare regulations, while a financial analyst must be familiar with financial markets and accounting principles.

Once the data has been analyzed, the next step is communicating the findings through reporting. Reporting involves presenting the insights in a format that is easy to understand and actionable for stakeholders. This can be done through various means, such as dashboards, charts, graphs, and written reports. The goal is to convey the key messages clearly and concisely, highlighting the most important findings and recommendations. Effective reporting can help stakeholders make informed decisions, track progress towards goals, and identify areas for improvement.

One of the key challenges in data analysis and reporting is ensuring data quality. Poor-quality data can lead to inaccurate analysis and misleading conclusions. Therefore, it is essential to implement robust data governance practices, including data validation, cleansing, and standardization. This ensures that the data used for analysis is accurate, complete, and consistent. Additionally, analysts must be aware of potential biases and limitations in the data and consider these when interpreting the results.

Another critical aspect of data analysis and reporting is using visualization techniques. Visualizations can make complex data more accessible and easier to understand. By representing data graphically, analysts can highlight trends, patterns, and outliers that may not be immediately apparent in raw data. Visualization techniques include bar charts, line graphs, scatter plots, and heat maps. The choice of visualization depends on the nature of the data and the specific insights that need to be communicated.

In addition to technical skills, practical data analysis and reporting require strong communication skills. Analysts must be able to explain their findings to non-technical stakeholders clearly and compellingly. This involves presenting the data and telling a story that connects the data to the organization's goals and objectives. By framing the insights within a broader narrative, analysts can help stakeholders understand the implications of the data and take appropriate actions.

The importance of data analysis and reporting cannot be overstated. In a competitive business environment, organizations that can harness the power of data are better positioned to succeed. Data-driven decision-making enables organizations to respond quickly to changing market conditions, identify new opportunities, and mitigate risks. It also fosters a culture of continuous improvement, as organizations can use data to measure performance, identify improvement areas, and track changes' impact over time.

To illustrate the impact of data analysis and reporting, consider the example of a retail company. By analyzing sales data, the company can identify which products are performing well and which are not. This information can be used to optimize inventory levels, adjust pricing strategies, and develop targeted marketing campaigns. Additionally, by analyzing customer data, the company can gain insights into customer preferences and behaviour, enabling them to personalize their offerings and improve customer satisfaction.

Data analysis and reporting can profoundly impact patient outcomes in the healthcare industry. Healthcare providers can identify trends and patterns that inform treatment decisions and improve patient care by analyzing patient data. For example, predictive analytics can identify patients at high risk of readmission, allowing providers to intervene early and prevent costly hospitalizations. Additionally, by analyzing data on treatment outcomes, providers can identify best practices and continuously improve the quality of care.

Data analysis and reporting are essential for managing risk and ensuring regulatory compliance in the financial sector. Financial institutions can use data analysis to detect fraudulent activities, assess credit risk, and monitor market trends. Effective reporting enables them to communicate these insights to regulators, investors, and other stakeholders, ensuring transparency and accountability.

In conclusion, data analysis and reporting are essential tools for organizations seeking to leverage the power of data. By transforming raw data into actionable insights and effectively communicating these insights, organizations can make informed decisions, optimize operations, and drive innovation. Analyzing and reporting data is a technical skill and a strategic advantage. Organizations that invest in building robust data analysis and reporting capabilities are better equipped to navigate the complexities of the modern business landscape.

Comprehensive Coding Case Studies

Case Study 1: E-commerce Platform Optimization

Background: An e-commerce company faced declining sales and customer engagement. Despite a robust product catalogue and competitive pricing, the platform struggled with high cart abandonment rates and low repeat purchase rates. The company decided to undertake a comprehensive analysis to identify and address the underlying issues.

Approach:

Data Collection: The team gathered data from various sources, including website analytics, customer feedback, transaction records, and user behaviour logs.

Data Cleaning: They cleaned the data to remove duplicates, correct errors, and fill in missing values.

Exploratory Data Analysis (EDA): The team conducted EDA to identify patterns and trends. They used visualizations to understand customer behaviour, such as heatmaps to track user interactions on the website.

Segmentation: Customers were segmented based on purchasing behaviour, demographics, and engagement levels. This helped identify distinct customer groups with unique needs and preferences.

Predictive Modeling: Machine learning models were developed to predict cart abandonment and customer churn. Features such as browsing history, time spent on the site, and previous purchase history were used in the models.

A/B Testing: Various website elements, such as the checkout process, product recommendations, and promotional offers, were tested to determine their impact on user behaviour.

Findings:

Cart Abandonment: The analysis revealed that a complex and lengthy checkout process significantly contributed to cart abandonment. Simplifying the checkout process and offering multiple payment options significantly reduced abandonment rates.

Customer Engagement: Personalized product recommendations and targeted email campaigns improved customer engagement and repeat purchase rates. Customers responded positively to recommendations based on their browsing and purchase history.

User Experience: Heatmaps showed that users struggled with navigation on mobile devices. Optimizing the mobile interface improved user experience and increased mobile sales.

Outcome: The e-commerce platform saw a 20% increase in sales and a 15% reduction in cart abandonment rates within six months. Customer satisfaction scores improved, and the company gained valuable insights into customer behaviour that informed future strategies.

Case Study 2: Healthcare Predictive Analytics

Background: A healthcare provider aimed to improve patient outcomes by leveraging predictive analytics. The goal was to identify patients at risk of readmission within 30 days of discharge and develop targeted interventions to prevent readmissions.

Approach:

Data Collection: The team collected data from electronic health records (EHRs), including patient demographics, medical history, treatment plans, and discharge summaries.

Data Cleaning: Data cleaning involves standardizing medical codes, handling missing values, and ensuring data consistency.

Feature Engineering: Relevant features were engineered from the raw data, such as the number of previous hospitalizations, comorbidities, medication adherence, and follow-up appointments.

Model Development: Various machine learning models, including logistic regression, decision trees, and random forests, were developed to predict readmission risk. The models were evaluated using metrics such as accuracy, precision, recall, and the area under the ROC curve (AUC-ROC).

Model Interpretation: Techniques such as SHAP (Shapley Additive exPlanations) were used to interpret the models and understand the factors contributing to readmission risk.

Intervention Design: Based on the model predictions, targeted interventions were designed, including follow-up calls, home visits, and personalized care plans.

Findings:

High-Risk Factors: The analysis identified critical factors associated with readmission risk, such as multiple chronic conditions, lack of follow-up care, and medication non-adherence.

Predictive Accuracy: The random forest model achieved the highest predictive accuracy, with an AUC-ROC of 0.85. This model was used to identify high-risk patients.

Intervention Impact: Targeted interventions for high-risk patients led to a significant reduction in readmission rates. Patients who received follow-up care and personalized support were less likely to be readmitted.

Outcome:

The healthcare provider achieved a 25% reduction in 30-day readmission rates. The predictive analytics approach improved patient outcomes and resulted in cost savings for the healthcare system. The insights gained from the analysis informed the development of proactive care strategies and enhanced patient management.

Case Study 3: Financial Fraud Detection

Background: A financial institution faced increasing fraudulent transactions, leading to significant economic losses and reputational damage. The institution sought to implement a robust fraud detection system using advanced analytics.

Approach:

Data Collection: Transaction data, including transaction amounts, timestamps, locations, and customer profiles, was collected. Historical fraud data was also included for model training.

Data Cleaning: The data was cleaned to remove noise, handle missing values, and ensure consistency.

Feature Engineering: Features such as transaction frequency, average transaction amount, and deviations from typical spending patterns were engineered to capture potential indicators of fraudulent activity.

Model Development: Various machine learning models, including logistic regression, support vector machines (SVM), and neural networks, were developed to detect fraudulent transactions. The models were trained on labelled data, with fraud and non-fraud transactions identified.

Model Evaluation: The models were evaluated using precision, recall, F1-score, and the area under the precision-recall curve (AUC-PR). Cross-validation techniques were employed to ensure the models' robustness and generalizability.

Real-Time Implementation: The best-performing model was integrated into the institution's transaction processing system to enable real-time fraud detection. Alerts were generated for transactions flagged as potentially fraudulent, allowing for immediate investigation and action.

Findings:

High-Risk Patterns: The analysis identified specific patterns associated with fraudulent transactions, such as unusually high transaction amounts, transactions occurring in quick succession, and transactions from geographically distant locations.

Model Performance: The neural network model outperformed other models, achieving a high F1-score and AUC-PR. This model was particularly effective in identifying subtle and complex patterns indicative of fraud.

Operational Efficiency: The real-time fraud detection system significantly reduced the time required to identify and respond to fraudulent transactions. The system's alerts enabled the institution to take swift action, minimizing financial losses and protecting customers.

Outcome: The financial institution experienced a 40% reduction in fraudulent transactions within the first three months of implementing the fraud detection system. Customer trust and satisfaction improved, and the institution's reputation was bolstered. The insights gained from the analysis also informed the development of enhanced security measures and fraud prevention strategies.

Case Study 4: Social Media Sentiment Analysis

Background: Analyzing social media data, a global brand sought to understand public sentiment towards its products and marketing campaigns. The goal was to gain insights into customer opinions, identify emerging trends, and inform marketing strategies.

Approach:

Data Collection: Social media data was collected from Twitter, Facebook, and Instagram. The data included posts, comments, likes, shares, and hashtags related to the brand and its products.

Data Cleaning: The data was cleaned to remove irrelevant content, spam, and duplicates. Text preprocessing techniques, such as tokenization, stemming, and stop-word removal, were applied to prepare the data for analysis.

Sentiment Analysis: Natural language processing (NLP) techniques were used for sentiment analysis. Models such as VADER (valence-aware dictionary and sentiment Reasoner) and BERT (Bidirectional Encoder Representations from Transformers) were employed to classify the sentiment of social media posts as positive, negative, or neutral.

Trend Analysis: Time-series analysis was conducted to identify trends in sentiment over time. The impact of specific events, such as product launches and marketing campaigns, on public sentiment was also analyzed.

Topic Modeling: Topic modelling techniques, such as Latent Dirichlet Allocation (LDA), were used to identify common themes and topics discussed by users. This provided insights into the aspects of the brand and the most essential products to customers.

Findings:

Sentiment Trends: The analysis revealed fluctuations in public sentiment corresponding to major events and marketing campaigns. Positive sentiment peaked during successful product launches, while negative sentiment spiked in response to product recalls and controversies.

Customer Insights: Topic modelling identified critical themes in customer discussions, such as product quality, customer service, and brand values. These insights helped the brand understand customer priorities and pain points.

Campaign Impact: The sentiment analysis provided valuable feedback on the effectiveness of marketing campaigns. Campaigns that resonated with customers and generated positive sentiment were identified, while those that received negative feedback were reevaluated.

Outcome:

The brand gained a deeper understanding of public sentiment and customer opinions. This informed the development of more targeted and effective marketing strategies. The insights from the sentiment analysis also guided product improvements and customer service enhancements, leading to increased customer satisfaction and loyalty.

Case Study 5: Predictive Maintenance in Manufacturing

Background: A manufacturing company aimed to reduce downtime and maintenance costs by implementing a predictive maintenance system. The goal was to predict equipment failures before they occurred and schedule maintenance proactively.

Approach:

Data Collection: Sensor data from manufacturing equipment, including temperature, vibration, pressure, and operational logs, was collected. Historical maintenance records and failure data were also included.

Data Cleaning: The data was cleaned to remove noise, handle missing values, and ensure consistency. Anomalies and outliers were carefully examined to distinguish between genuine issues and sensor errors.

Feature Engineering: Relevant features were engineered from the raw sensor data, such as moving averages, standard deviations, and frequency domain features. These features captured the operational characteristics of the equipment.

Model Development: Machine learning models, including time series, random forests, and gradient-boosting machines, were developed to predict equipment failures. The models were trained on historical data, with failure events clearly labelled.

Model Evaluation: The models were evaluated using metrics such as precision, recall, F1-score, and the area under the receiver operating characteristic curve (AUC-ROC). Cross-validation techniques ensured the models' robustness and generalizability.

Real-Time Implementation: The best-performing model was integrated into the manufacturing company's monitoring system. Real-time predictions of equipment failures were generated, allowing for proactive maintenance scheduling.

Findings:

Failure Patterns: The analysis identified specific patterns and conditions associated with equipment failures, such as abnormal temperature spikes, increased vibration levels, and irregular pressure readings.

Model Performance: The gradient boosting machine model outperformed other models, achieving a high F1-score and AUC-ROC. This model was particularly effective in capturing complex interactions between different sensor readings.

Operational Efficiency: The predictive maintenance system significantly reduced unplanned downtime and maintenance costs. The system's predictions enabled the company to schedule maintenance activities during planned downtimes, minimizing disruptions to production.

Outcome: The manufacturing company experienced a 30% reduction in unplanned downtime and a 25% decrease in maintenance costs within the first six months of implementing the predictive maintenance system. The improved reliability of equipment operations led to increased production efficiency and reduced operational risks. The insights gained from the analysis also informed the development of more effective maintenance strategies and practices.

Case Study 6: Customer Churn Prediction

Background: A telecommunications company aimed to reduce customer churn by predicting which customers were likely to leave and implementing targeted retention strategies. The goal was to improve customer retention rates and increase long-term revenue.

Approach:

Data Collection: Customer data, including demographic information, service usage patterns, billing history, and customer support interactions, was collected. Historical churn data was also included.

Data Cleaning: The data was cleaned to handle missing values, remove duplicates, and ensure consistency. Outliers and anomalies were carefully examined to distinguish between genuine issues and data errors.

Feature Engineering: Relevant features were engineered from the raw customer data, such as average monthly usage, billing consistency, and frequency of customer support interactions. These features captured the behavioral characteristics of customers.

Model Development: Machine learning models, including logistic regression, decision trees, and random forests, were developed to predict customer churn. The models were trained on historical data, with churn events clearly labeled.

Model Evaluation: The models were evaluated using metrics such as precision, recall, F1-score, and the area under the receiver operating characteristic curve (AUC-ROC). Cross-validation techniques ensured the models' robustness and generalizability.

Targeted Retention Strategies: The best-performing model was used to identify high-risk customers. Targeted retention strategies, such as personalized offers, loyalty programs, and proactive customer support, were implemented to retain these customers.

Findings

Churn Patterns: The analysis identified specific patterns and behaviors associated with customer churns, such as declining service usage, inconsistent billing payments, and frequent negative interactions with customer support.

Model Performance: The random forest model outperformed other models, achieving a high F1-score and AUC-ROC. This model was particularly effective in capturing complex interactions between different customer behaviors.

Retention Strategies: The targeted retention strategies significantly reduced customer churn rates. Personalized offers and loyalty programs were particularly effective in retaining high-risk customers.

Outcome: The telecommunications company experienced a 20% reduction in customer churn rates within the first year of implementing the churn prediction system. The improved customer retention rates increased long-term revenue and enhanced customer satisfaction. The insights gained from the analysis also informed the development of more effective customer engagement and retention strategies.

EXTRA CONTENTS

Audiobook

The audiobook version of Medical Billing & Coding Mastery in 4 Months adds significant value by allowing you to conveniently learn and review essential concepts on the go, transforming commute or workout time into productive training sessions and providing an engaging, interactive way to master exam strategies and job-hunting tactics.

Full Additional Video Course (100+ Video)

The Full Additional Video Course (100+ videos) included significantly enhances the learning experience by offering visual and interactive content that simplifies complex topics, ensuring a deeper understanding and retention of essential skills, while providing practical insights and real-world applications to better prepare you for exams and job searches.

Find A Job In 4 Months! - The Best 10 Opportunities To Discover

The Find A Job In 4 Months! - The Best 10 Opportunities To Discover bonus included provides invaluable guidance by highlighting top job prospects in the field, streamlining your job search and significantly increasing your chances of securing a rewarding position quickly and efficiently.

Download And Print - Exercise With Our Medical Journal!

The Download And Print - Exercise With Our Medical Journal! bonus included adds substantial value by providing hands-on practice opportunities.

300+ Digital Flashcards

The 300+ Digital Flashcards bonus included with Medical Billing & Coding Mastery in 4 Months significantly enhances your study efficiency by offering a convenient and effective way to review and memorize key concepts, ensuring you can quickly recall important information and excel in both exams and professional settings.

Ebook Medical Terminology With 1500+ Key Terms | 600 Questions And Answers | 400+ Digital Flashcards

The Ebook Medical Terminology With 1500+ Key Terms | 600 Questions And Answers | 400+ Digital Flashcards bonus included with Medical Billing & Coding Mastery in 4 Months greatly enriches your learning experience by providing extensive resources to master medical terminology, test your knowledge, and reinforce your understanding through interactive flashcards, ensuring you are thoroughly prepared for both exams and real-world applications.

Scan the QR CODE that is on the page below

Made in United States
Cleveland, OH
15 February 2025

14384588R00077